THE B VITAMINS

How these vitamins function, what happens when they
are grossly and mildly deficient, how they can help as
therapeutic agents in many disorders, and which foods
we should eat to ensure an adequate supply.

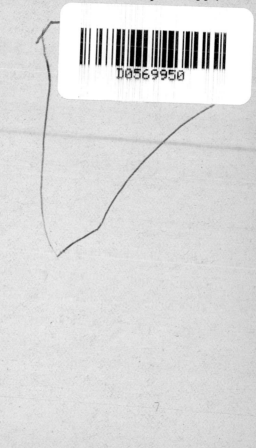

THE B VITAMINS

Their Major Role in Maintaining Your Health

by

LEONARD MERVYN
B.Sc., Ph.D., F.R.S.C.

NATURE'S WAY

THORSONS PUBLISHERS INC.
New York

Thorsons Publishers Inc.
377 Park Avenue South
New York, New York 10016

First U.S. Edition 1983

© LEONARD MERVYN 1981

LIBRARY OF CONGRESS CATALOGING IN PUBLICATION DATA

Mervyn, Len
  The B vitamins.
  Includes index.
  1. Vitamin B complex — Physiological effect
  2. Vitamin B in human nutrition.   3. Vitamin B complex—
  Therapeutic use   I. Title.
QP772.V52M47   1983   613.2'8   83-5051
ISBN 0-7225-0667-8

Printed in Great Britain by
Richard Clay (The Chaucer Press) Ltd., Bungay, Suffolk

Thorsons Publishers Inc. are distributed to the trade by
Inner Traditions International Ltd., New York

CONTENTS

This book is lovingly dedicated to
my wife Beryl.

INTRODUCTION

Strictly speaking, a substance can be regarded as a true vitamin only if it satisfies three criteria. First, it cannot be made by body tissues and must be obtained from the food. Second, when it is deficient in the body certain clinical and biochemical symptoms manifest themselves. Third, these symptoms and signs of deficiency are reversed by treatment with the appropriate vitamin.

When we look at the vitamin B-complex in terms of these criteria, it becomes obvious that only certain members of the complex are true B vitamins. The others, although invariably accompanying the true vitamins in foods and in the body cannot strictly be regarded as vitamins. This in no way decries their importance to health, but since the food is not their sole source it means that daily requirements are impossible to assess. This fact assumes great importance when, later in the book, we discuss the therapeutic application of some members of the complex.

Categorizing B vitamins

At present, the vitamin B-complex comprises fourteen

known factors, all characterized by their solubility in water. Eight of them must be regarded as true vitamins on the basis of the above criteria, and they are: B_1 – thiamine; B_2 – riboflavin; B_6 – pyridoxine; B_{12} – cyanocobalamin; pantothenic acid; nicotinamide; biotin and folic acid. The designation of a B-number for some of these vitamins goes back to the days of their discovery when as each was isolated it was given a number, since the chemical structure was not known until later. At first, all these B vitamins were assumed to be a group of chemical compounds called 'amines' hence the ending 'amine' on many of them. This false assumption was later disproved but the names stuck.

Although the practice of numbering the B vitamins continues until this day, there is now a trend away from it, and for very good reasons. For example, vitamin B_3 refers to nicotinic acid (or its alternatives) in the U.S.A., but in Europe B_3 is regarded as pantothenic acid. Conversely, in the U.S.A. B_5 is designated pantothenic acid, while in Europe B_5 is regarded as the nicotinic acid group. This sort of confusion does not arise if names are used, and it is strongly recommended that labels and literature should carry at least the names of the B vitamins, with the numbers only as additional information.

The exception in the above eight true vitamins is nicotinic acid, which can in fact be made by body tissues from an essential precursor called L-tryptophan, a constituent of proteins. The amounts made this way, however, are too small to fulfil the body's daily requirements for the vitamin and an extraneous supply is still necessary. On the other hand, it is likely that three other members of the B-complex, choline, inositol and orotic acid, can be manufactured in adequate amounts by a healthy individual. Para-aminobenzoic acid (PABA) is an essential B vitamin for bacteria but, even though it has not been shown to be necessary for man and animals, it is certainly a member of the B-complex. The remaining two members are pangamic acid, known also as B_{15} (or, incorrectly, as vitamin B_{15}) and laetrile or B_{17} (or, incorrectly, as vitamin B_{17}). The importance of the last six members mentioned lies in their therapeutic application in certain complaints and these will be discussed later in the book.

The Missing Numbers

People often wonder what happened to the missing numbers of the B-complex. During the heady days when the vitamins were being discovered, research groups often designated a compound as a B vitamin, gave it a number then later found that it was not a vitamin at all. For example, vitamin B_4 was found to be adenine, a compound of profound importance in the body which, however, can be synthesized by the body in *adequate* amounts. Similarly, vitamins B_7, B_8 and B_9 were found to be essential growth factors for micro-organisms that had no counterparts in man. Vitamins B_{10} and B_{11} were claimed to be growth factors for chicks but were never characterized. Vitamin B_{14} turned out to be a simple derivative of vitamin B_{12} and so became part of the widespread group of B_{12} vitamins.

Table 1 sums up the various members of the B-complex with their designations and alternative names.

B-complex Functions

The B-complex functions in the body as a group of vitamins, each dependent upon the others. They are essential in the production of energy from food and vital for the metabolism of fats and protein. Correct functioning of the brain and nervous system requires an adequate supply of the B-complex. They are necessary in maintaining an efficient digestive system. The group as a whole contribute to healthy skin, hair, eyes, mouth and liver. The production of haemoglobin, the red pigment in blood that carries oxygen to the muscles and organs of the body, is under the control of some of the members of the B-complex.

Vitamin B Deficiency

All of the B vitamins, with the possible exception of B_{12}, are natural constituents of brewer's yeast, liver, wholegrain

Table 1. Members of the Vitamin B-Complex

Common Name	Alternative Names	Number	Supplement Form
Thiamine	Aneurine	B_1	Hydrochloride; Nitrate.
Riboflavin	Lactoflavine Vitamin G	B_2	Phosphate.
Nicotinamide	Niacinamide Vitamin PP	B_3 (U.S.A.) B_5 (Europe)	As free vitamin; ascorbate.
Nicotinic Acid	Niacin PP Factor	B_3 (U.S.A.) B_5 (Europe)	As free vitamin.
Pantothenic Acid	Chick Antidermatitis Factor	B_5 (U.S.A.) B_3 (Europe)	Calcium pantothenate.
Pyridoxine Pyridoxal Pyridoxamine	none	B_6 B_6 B_6	Hydrochloride; Phosphate.
Cyanocobalamin Hydroxocobalamin	Extrinsic Factor LLD Factor Anti-Pernicious Anaemia Factor	B_{12} $B_{12}a$; $B_{12}b$	As free vitamin; Hydrochloride; Acetate.
Folic Acid	Vitamin Bc; PGA; Vitamin M	—	As free vitamin.
Folinic Acid	Citrovorum Factor	—	Calcium folinate.
Biotin	Vitamin H Bios II	—	As free vitamin.
Choline	Amanitine	—	Bitartrate; Chloride.
Inositol	Bios I Myo-Inositol Meso-Inositol	—	As free compound; Niacinate.
Para-aminobenzoic Acid	PABA Vitamin Bx Bacterial Vitamin H Anti-grey Hair Factor (rats)	—	As free compound.
Orotic Acid	Whey Factor Animal Galactose Factor	B_{13}	As free compound; Choline orotate.
Pangamic Acid		B_{15}	Calcium pangamate; Sodium pangamate.
Laetrile	Amygdalin	B_{17}	Powdered apricot kernel.

cereals and green vegetables. Although a full, well-balanced diet should give adequate quantities of the whole complex, there are many factors that can contribute to destruction of some of the members. Cooking, bad storage of food, food refining and processing, habits like smoking tobacco and drinking alcoholic beverages and prolonged use of the contraceptive pill can all cause deficiency to varying degrees of the components of the B-complex. Some medicinal drugs can induce specific deficiencies when taken over a long period. Since the vitamins are all water-soluble, the body has no way of storing them and an adequate daily intake is essential.

If there is doubt about the adequacy of the daily intake from food, it is possible to ensure ample quantities by taking B-complex supplements. It is important to remember to take all the B vitamins together because they are so interrelated in function that, apart from some special circumstances, a simple deficiency in one of them is unlikely. Natural forms of the B vitamins are preferable to the synthetic ones since they may contain other factors, as yet unknown, that would not accompany those synthesized in a laboratory.

The need for the B-complex increases during stress situations, including those produced by infection. The body usually responds to stress conditions by increasing its production of hormones to overcome the effects of stress. These hormones cannot be manufactured without the aid of the B-complex. Hence the benefit that often results from a supplemental intake of the B-complex during times of stress, remembering also that vitamin C taken with it is extra helpful. Stress diseases such as arthritis are helped in a similar fashion.

What happens when a person is deficient in the B complex? What sort of symptoms would one expect? Tiredness, irritability, nervous symptoms, and mild depression are amongst the most common. Grey hair, loss of hair, acne, psoriasis, eczema, and other skin problems may be related to a lack of the B-group. A poor appetite, insomnia, lethargy, anaemia, and constipation can all result from deficiency of the B-complex. At the same time many of these symptoms will respond to supplementation with the whole complex.

Responsive Conditions

The medical literature is full of examples of ailments that have responded to treatment with the B-complex. These include Ménière's Syndrome, a disease of the inner ear characterized by recurrent attacks of deafness, ringing in the ears (tinnitus), vertigo, nausea and vomiting. Migraine headaches can be controlled with high doses of the B-complex. Mental deterioration in very old people will often be halted by the B vitamins and mental ability is often restored. Children are now treated with high potency B-complex for schizophrenia, hyperactivity, aggressiveness and other psychological conditions. Shingles appears to respond favourably to the B-group. Mild depression can often be overcome with B vitamins, particularly vitamin B_6, where the condition has been precipitated by drugs. The complex can have a calming effect and so induce sleep where insomnia is due to anxiety. The vitamin B-complex has been used with success in treating menstrual problems, including premenstrual tension. Those at the menopause will often benefit by supplementation.

The B-complex may be taken with advantage in those suffering from heart disease. The vitamins help by ensuring that blood fats are kept in solution and blood cholesterol is kept down to normal levels to reduçe the chances of a thrombosis forming. At the same time the nerves controlling the heart need the B-complex for smooth, quiet functioning.

To sum up, it can be stated that the vitamin B-complex controls such a wide range of body functions that whenever anything goes wrong, the B-group can often be beneficial. In the chapters that follow we shall see how these vitamins function, what happens when they are mildly and grossly deficient, how they can help as safe therapeutic agents in many disorders and which foods should we eat to ensure an adequate daily supply.

1
THE ENERGY VITAMINS

The first three members of the vitamin B-complex, thiamine, riboflavin and nicotinamide are related through their functions in converting the food we eat into the energy we need. Carbohydrates, fats and proteins are the constituents of food that give rise to energy, but the conversion relies upon reactions that are completely dependent upon these three vitamins. Energy production is not confined to muscles but is essential for every living process, including circulation of the blood, functioning of the digestive system and maintenance of a healthy brain and nervous system.

The history of how the presence of these vitamins was first suspected and their subsequent isolation and identification represents a fascinating story of observation and persistence. It also illustrates the importance of relating the symptoms of a human deficiency disease with those in animals, since the latter then represent an ideal model on which to carry out further research.

Thiamine (Vitamin B$_1$)
In 1885, a Japanese naval surgeon, K. Takaki, was the first to

demonstrate that the disease known as beri beri in man was associated with an excessive intake of polished rice in the diet. He was able to reduce the incidence of the disease in either of two ways: (a) by replacing part of the rice in the ration by wheaten bread and increasing the intake of vegetables and milk; or (b) by simply replacing polished rice with the unpolished variety that contained the husk. Parallel studies on domestic fowls by the Dutch physician C. Eijkman in 1897 indicated that feeding these birds polished rice induced a disease with symptoms similar to beri beri. This disease, too, was reversed by including rice husk and germ in the bird's diet. However, it was not until 1926 that Doctors B. C. P. Jansen and W. F. Donath working in Eijkman's laboratory succeeded in isolating the factor from rice polishings that prevented beri beri. Hence the vitamin thiamine was discovered.

What Does Thiamine Do?

Glucose is converted into energy via a compound known as pyruvic acid. Thiamine is responsible for ensuring that this pyruvic acid is fed into the energy cycle. Hence, in the absence of thiamine, pyruvic acid accumulates in the body and high blood levels result. This reaction represents only one of the twenty-five or so functions that thiamine performs in a healthy body but, when things go wrong, it is the easiest to detect. High blood pyruvic acid levels give rise to an oxygen deficiency that results in loss of mental alertness, respiratory problems and heart damage. The early symptoms of thiamine deficiency, therefore, include easy fatigue, anorexia (loss of appetite), nausea, muscle weakness and digestive upsets. Emotional disturbances are also observed including depression and irritability with impairment of memory and the powers of concentration. These symptoms reflect the dependence of the nervous system on glucose as its main source of energy.

A high blood pyruvic acid level has more sinister manifestations. It causes blood vessels to dilate to an extreme degree allowing fluid to leak into the surrounding tissues to produce oedema (swelling). In an attempt to maintain the blood circulation, the heart steps up its output, but heart muscle itself needs thiamine for efficient functioning and so it finds it difficult to meet the extra demands upon it. This vicious circle continues until heart failure is the eventual result.

The symptoms and sequence of events mentioned describe what happens in beri beri which is related to a gross deficiency of thiamine. However even a mild deficiency of the vitamin can give rise to symptoms. Early symptoms are commonplace and include such non-specific complaints as fatigue, weight-loss and anorexia. The person lacks energy and is constantly tired; he does not sleep well and appears irritable. As deficiency worsens, the memory becomes faulty and the concentration poor. The individual becomes unstable emotionally, over-reacting to normal stresses and strains. He is constipated with vague abdominal and chest pains. Eventually the nervous symptoms get worse resulting in a tingling and burning in the toes and soles of his feet and the calves become extremely tender.

These results were noted in healthy volunteers who deliberately withheld thiamine from their diets. The earliest sign of deficiency was nausea and this appeared only three to seven days after complete deprivation. From then on, however, there was a definite correlation between the extent of the various symptoms and the lack of thiamine. What was particularly disturbing was that the effects on the brain and nervous system resulting in personality changes appeared long before the more obvious symptoms like gastrointestinal distress, loss of appetite and loss in weight.

The Growth Vitamin

Vitamin B_1 is also required for growth. German studies reported in 1977 found that 11 per cent of the pregnant women studied had borderline body levels of the vitamin during the first three months of pregnancy. These women invariably gave birth to babies of low birth weight. Perinatal mortality increases as birth-weight decreases, so it is important to ensure an adequate intake of thiamine during pregnancy.

There is no need to feel complacent in the Western world about our intake of vitamin B_1. G. B. Brubacher in a recent symposium on 'The Importance of Vitamins to Human Health' (IV Kellogg Nutrition Symposium, 1978) concluded that, 'in modern society, as a consequence of eating habits and lack of exercise, vitamin B_1 will be one of the nutrients which will become or may even be already a limiting factor in the nutrition of the general population'. A study reported in the *American Journal of Clinical Nutrition* (March, 1977) found that almost half the patients in nursing homes and elderly residents of private homes received less than two-thirds of their thiamine requirements in their diets. Bio-chemical evidence of vitamin B_1 deficiency is relatively common amongst the elderly in whom it may be associated with mental confusion. How can such deficiencies arise?

Dietary Losses of Thiamine
Thiamine is the most unstable member of the B-complex and is readily destroyed by alkaline conditions, particularly in the presence of copper. Alkaline baking powder can cause up to 50 per cent loss of flour thiamine; the use of soda when boiling vegetables is likely to destroy most of the vitamin present. Complete destruction of thiamine occurs with sulphur dioxide, often used as a preservative in foods like minced meat. All cooking methods destroy some vitamin B_1 and losses are low in braising and broiling techniques, but high in dry canning of meats.

By far the largest losses of thiamine are due to its solubility in water, although the vitamin may be reclaimed by consumption of the cooking water. Potatoes represent the only vegetable to make a significant contribution to the dietary intake of thiamine, so any processing with water will leach out the vitamin. Dipping potatoes in sulphite solution is carried out to retain their white colour in ready-peeled potatoes and potato crisps, but the process destroys up to 60 per cent of the thiamine, and subsequent storage and further cooking removes most of the remainder. Even careful cooking of an ordinary mixed diet starting with raw foods will result in losses of 25 per cent of the thiamine.

Other Factors Causing Thiamine Loss

Vitamin B_1 is concerned with the oxidation of carbohydrate. Hence it is important to maintain an intake of the vitamin that is related to that of carbohydrate, and this has been proposed as 0.096mg thiamine per 240 kilocalories (1 megajoule). This means that 1.5mg should be regarded as the daily minimum intake for most people, unless they are on a high refined carbohydrate diet.

Excessive consumption of refined carbohydrates can induce a deficiency of thiamine because these foods have had their vitamin removed during processing and refining. The balance is upset and the mild deficiency symptoms mentioned above may appear. Pregnancy, lactation, fever, surgery and other stressful conditions also call for an increased intake of thiamine, as does increased physical activity. Older people appear to have a greater need for thiamine. A clinical trial reported in *The Sciences* (1968) compared a group of women aged 19 to 21 with that of a group 52 to 75 years of age, with respect to their daily use of the vitamin. Despite the same intake, the older group excreted less. When deprived of the vitamin the older group exhibited adverse symptoms much more quickly. Such results suggest a greater need by the elderly for vitamin B_1 or they may simply reflect less efficient absorption by this group. Whatever the reason, the simplest measure is to ensure adequate intake in the elderly either by sensible diets or by supplementation.

Alcohol can exert a deleterious effect upon the body levels of thiamine. Lowered blood levels of the vitamin were reported in alcohol drinkers in the *Journal of Laboratory and Clinical Medicine* (1970). The studies indicated that alcohol interfered with vitamin B_1 utilization by the liver, preventing the conversion of thiamine to its active form. Alcohol also inhibits absorption of the vitamin from the food. The importance of thiamine in detoxifying alcohol has been underlined by Dr H. Sprince and his team from the Veterans Administration Hospital, Pennsylvania. Most alcohol drunk is converted first to a poisonous substance called acetaldehyde which is also present in tobacco smoke. The best combination to dispose of this material is thiamine, vitamin C and an amino acid known as L-cysteine. Tragically therefore, the very B vitamin required to rid the body of acetaldehyde produced either from alcohol or from tobacco smoke, is thiamine which is already in low supply in those partaking of these habits. Official concern about vitamin B_1 deficiency in alcohol drinkers has now reached such proportions that there are at present attempts in many countries to introduce legislation making supplementation of wines and spirits with the vitamin compulsory.

Prolonged taking of proprietary antacid preparations, particularly amongst the older group (but also amongst younger people who suffer from persistent dyspepsia), is another habit that can lead to impaired absorption of thiamine with subsequent low body levels of the vitamin.

Ensuring an Adequate Intake of Vitamin B_1

All animal and plant foods contain thiamine, but there is wide variation in their content. The germs of cereals, potatoes, nuts, peas, beans and other pulses are particularly rich. All green vegetables, root vegetables, fruits, fresh food and dairy products (except butter) supply the vitamin, but only at low concentrations. Organ meats such as liver, kidney and heart are much richer sources than muscle meats. Yeast and yeast extracts are particularly good sources of the vitamin. Natural foods are a more wholesome source of thiamine – for example brown rice contains 2.93mg per 100g compared to only 0.6mg per 100g in white rice. Even enriched white flour contains 30 per cent less thiamine than wholewheat flour. The more important food sources of thiamine are given in Table 2 (see page 26).

It must be remembered, however, that losses due to smoking, drinking and antacids may be more than can even be obtained from a good diet, and those who partake of these habits may have to seek extra intake from dietary supplements.

Conditions Where Thiamine May Help

When we consider how essential thiamine is to nerve and brain function, it is perhaps not surprising that the vitamin appears to improve mental ability. In a study of children aged 9 to 19 years, Dr R. F. Harvell of Columbia University compared the effect of supplementation with the relatively low level of 2 mg thiamine per day on one group with that of an unsupplemented group. Diets in both groups were identical and thought to be adequate. After one year's trial there was a large increase in the mental achievements of those receiving the extra vitamin using the criteria of mental alertness, emotional stability, lack of depression and zest for life. Neither group at any time showed symptoms of B_1 deficiency suggesting that the added vitamin was exerting an effect over and above that of the norm.

Those who suffer from the excessive attentions of insects can be helped by vitamin B_1 according to a report in *Medical Letters* (1968). Out of 100 sufferers in one trial, more than 70 per cent reported that on a daily intake of 75 to 100 mg daily, insects bothered them little or not at all. It is highly unlikely that at this level of intake the thiamine is acting in its true vitamin role, but rather as a therapeutic internal insect repellent. No side-effects were noted in this trial.

Thiamine is essential for a healthy heart. Dr J. B. Sutherland of the University of Ottawa School of Medicine found that lack of vitamin B_1 in rats caused slowed heart-beats, enlarged hearts and eventual heart failure. These findings were related to a heavy dependence of the heart on the vitamin for its energy production. In man, studies reported in *Nutrition Reviews* (October, 1955) revealed that the thiamine contents of heart muscle from those patients dying of heart failure were lower than those who had healthy diets but had died from other causes. The most likely cause was felt to be a prolonged inadequate intake of the vitamin in the patient's diet. This conclusion was also reached by Professor E. Cheraskin writing in the *Journal of the American Geriatrics Society* (1967) who studied the problem from a different approach. He measured the intakes of thiamine in healthy human beings, then followed their medical history. Those with the lower intakes ended up with twice the number of heart problems of those taking the higher amounts in their food. An extension of this trial revealed that the lower intake of the vitamin B_1 was associated with a higher intake of refined carbohydrate. This was felt to be the prime factor in the development of a mild deficiency of vitamin B_1.

Thiamine is perfectly safe when given orally in amounts totalling hundreds of milligrams. Occasional toxicity has been reported, but only when the vitamin was given intramuscularly or intravenously by injection.

Riboflavin (Vitamin B_2)

The discovery of riboflavin is typical of the way in which divergent researches on the same vitamin resulted in its ultimate characterization. Although known as a pigment of milk since 1879, it was not until 1928 that Dr R. Kuhn and his group in Germany investigated its growth-promoting properties and reported a heat-stable vitamin that they designated vitamin B_2. Experimental rats did not grow without this particular factor so, by using the rat as a measuring system, they were able to isolate the active principle; 1g of pure yellow material from 5,400 litres of whey. At about the same time, Dr O. Warburg and his research team had discovered a so-called 'yellow-enzyme' in yeast that was essential for cell respiration. This contained the same yellow compound that had been isolated from milk. What was a growth factor for both rats and yeast was soon realized also to be essential for man, and so the vitamin riboflavin was discovered.

Riboflavin is described as a heat-stable vitamin, but this is only true in acid solution. In the presence of alkali it is readily destroyed by heat. Light, however, is the great destroyer of riboflavin, particularly in milk. Milk sold under the strong lights of supermarkets in glass bottles can lose its riboflavin in 20 minutes. Packing milk in opaque cartons makes the vitamin far more stable. Even bread has been known to lose riboflavin, when wrapped in clear plastic and exposed to light.

One tragic consequence of the destruction of riboflavin by light is that the resulting product called lumiflavin itself destroys vitamin C. As little as 5 per cent lumiflavin, which is inactive as a vitamin, will destroy half the vitamin C present. The consequences of leaving milk in sunlight or artificial light can thus be imagined. The only obvious sign that milk has been exposed in this way is an off-taste termed 'sunlight flavour'.

Hence, in the absence of light and alkali, riboflavin is stable to most cooking methods. Like the other members of the B-complex however the greatest losses in cooking occur because of leaching into the cooking fluids or juices. Consumption of these in one form or another will ensure that such losses are reclaimed.

Riboflavin has a strong yellow colour, and in light its solution fluoresces, even at very low concentration. After taking the vitamin in tablets or capsules, the urine is often a highly-hued yellow colour. This may be disconcerting to the individual, but is in fact completely harmless as it is merely the body's way of excreting excess riboflavin. At least it proves that the vitamin has been absorbed.

The Function of Riboflavin

The importance of riboflavin stems from its integral roles when attached to certain specific proteins. Both riboflavin (known as the coenzyme) and the protein (known as the enzyme) combine and accelerate a large number of body reactions without which life would be impossible. There are two of these combinations in the body known as FMN (flavin mononucleotide) and FAD (flavin adenine dinucleotide) and riboflavin is common to both although the protein differs. One fundamental role of these riboflavin-protein combinations is in the oxidation of amino acids (from protein), fatty acids (from fats) and sugars (from carbohydrates), the energy-producing constituents of food. Riboflavin is essential for body cell respiration to ensure efficient utilization of oxygen. The vitamin is necessary for the production and repair of body tissues and appears to have a particular function in maintaining healthy mucous membranes, the moist surfaces of the body. Hence the eyes and mouth are usually the first to suffer in the early stages of riboflavin deficiency. The vitamin riboflavin is necessary in the conversion of tryptophan to nicotinic acid but this only has importance when dietary intake of nicotinic acid is low.

Riboflavin Deficiency

Riboflavin deficiency in young animals results in a failure to grow, but there are many manifestations that are also exhibited in adults. These include impaired reproduction with congenital malformations in the offspring. Anaemia sometimes occurs since riboflavin is needed for red blood cell production. Skin conditions induced by deficiency include dermatitis, and an unhealthy scalp, leading to hair loss. The most serious complaints involve the eyes of animals resulting in conjunctivitis, bloodshot eyes and cataract. The inability to metabolize fat gives rise to fatty livers.

Similar lesions were observed in riboflavin deficiency in man when this was induced in volunteers in a trial reported by W. H. Sebrell and R. E. Butler in *Public Health Reports* (Washington, 1938). After a period of four months when the subjects received only 0.5mg vitamin B_2 per day, they developed cracks and sores in the corner of the mouth with inflammation of the tongue and lips. The eyes were badly affected becoming bloodshot and developing a burning sensation with a feeling of grit and sand on the insides of the eyelids. There was increased sensitivity to light and the eyes became easily fatigued. Skin changes occurred with scaling around the nose, mouth, forehead and ears; the scalp was affected in a similar manner leading to excessive hair loss.

Despite the occasional appearance of trembling, dizziness, insomnia and a slow mental attitude in B_2 deficiency, the vitamin does not appear to be as important to the mental system as the other B vitamins.

Avoiding Deficiency

Dietary habits are the most likely reason for a low intake of riboflavin, whether due to eating the wrong foods, poor cooking techniques, specialized diets that may miss out riboflavin-rich foods (e.g. milk and dairy-free diets), restricted diets taken in gastro-intestinal complaints. Alcoholism can give rise to vitamin B_2 deficiency, but this is more a generalized low intake of the B-complex rather than a specific lack of B_2. Amongst drugs in common use, the contraceptive pill is the only one likely to lead to low body levels of the vitamin. The abnormality probably results from the oestrogenic component, but the mechanism involved is not certain. Supplementation with vitamin B_2 represents the simplest way to overcome this problem, preferably at a level of 10mg per day.

The most important foods containing vitamin B_2 are liver, milk, products made from milk, eggs and green vegetables. Yeast and yeast extracts are particularly rich sources. Unlike the other members of the vitamin B-complex, grains, flours and cereals do not contain much riboflavin naturally, although fortification has helped to redress the balance. Beer is a good source of the vitamin but excessive intake may allow the alcohol content to have a deleterious effect upon the body levels of riboflavin. Table 2 gives the riboflavin content of various food items. A good diet will ensure the recommended minimum intake of 2mg per day.

Therapeutic Uses of Riboflavin

Riboflavin at high doses has been tried in a number of diseases, but the success is rather variable when compared to the positive therapeutic effect associated with some other members of the vitamin B-complex. Recurrent mouth

Table 2.
The Energy Vitamins in Raw Foods (mg per 100g)

Food Item	Thiamine (Vit.B_1)	Riboflavin (Vit.B_2)	Nicotinic Acid (Total)*
Liver (pig)	0.31	3.0	19.4
Kidney (pig)	0.32	1.9	11.0
Beef	0.07	0.24	9.5
Lamb	0.14	0.28	10.4
Pork	0.89	0.25	10.0
Chicken	0.10	0.16	11.6
Fish (white)	0.08	0.07	4.9
Fish (fatty)	0.20	0.15	10.4
Eggs (whole)	0.09	0.47	3.7
Milk (cows)	0.04	0.19	0.86
Cheese (hard)	0.04	0.50	6.2
Cheese (cottage)	0.02	0.19	3.3
Yogurt	0.05	0.26	1.2
Wholemeal bread	0.26	0.06	5.6
White bread	0.18	0.03	3.0
Wheat bran	0.89	0.36	32.6
Wheatgerm	2.00	0.68	4.2
Wheat grains	0.46	0.08	8.1
Oatflakes	0.55	0.14	4.1
Maize (corn)	0.20	0.06	1.0
Rice (unpolished, brown)	2.93	0.05	4.7
Soya flour (full fat)	0.75	0.31	10.6
Citrus fruits (peeled)	0.10	0.03	0.3
Dried fruits	0.07	0.19	5.6
Bananas	0.04	0.07	0.8
Nuts (fresh)	0.90	0.10	21.3
Nuts (roasted)	0.23	0.10	21.3
Potatoes	0.11	0.04	1.7
Root vegetables (carrots etc.)	0.06	0.05	0.7
Greenleaf vegetables	0.06	0.25	0.8
Pulses (beans, peas etc.)	0.32	0.15	3.4
Yeast (brewer's, dried)	15.6	4.3	37.9
Yeast extract	3.1	11.0	67.0
Honey	0.01	0.05	0.2

*Figure refers to free nicotinic acid plus that derived from tryptophan.

ulcers have been claimed to be prevented by daily intakes of 20mg or more of vitamin B_2. Similar studies on stomach and duodenal ulcers resulted in a less dramatic response, but this was probably because these lesions are a result of many factors amongst which may be riboflavin deficiency.

Ulceration of the cornea of the eye will sometimes respond to high potency supplementation with vitamin B_2. In a study of 47 patients suffering from eye and eyesight problems, six of whom were affected by cataracts, Dr U. P. Sydenstricker reported in *Prevention* (November, 1970) that all disorders were gradually cured with vitamin B_2 supplementation. It was essential to carry on with the high riboflavin intake since, when this ceased, the eye complaints returned.

These results parallel those in animals suffering from this condition, but it must be stressed that other B vitamins, like pantothenic acid, may also be involved in prevention of cataracts.

According to I. Stockley in *Drug Interactions and their Mechanisms* (Pharmaceutical Press, 1974), riboflavin almost never causes adverse reactions. In fact, the vitamin is considered so safe that it is accepted as a natural colouring agent that may be added to foods.

Nicotinic Acid (Nicotinamide)

The compound nicotinic acid has been known to organic chemists since 1867, but then it was merely regarded as an interesting chemical substance. It was not until 1913 that Dr C. Funk showed that it occurred naturally in foods and isolated the compound from yeast and rice polishings. His aim was in finding a cure for beri beri and when nicotinic acid did not help in the disease, interest in the acid was lost. At about the same time in the U.S.A., Dr J. Goldberger of the U.S. Public Health Service was given the task of finding out what caused the disease pellagra which at that time was rife in the southern states of America. By a combination of epidemiological studies (occurrence and distribution of disease) and experimental studies, Dr Goldberger was able to demonstrate that pellagra was a deficiency disease associated with the poor diets that were prevalent in the affected areas at the time. He was able to cure the disease by providing supplements of yeast, lean beef and milk, but although he postulated that the curative factor was a member of the vitamin B-complex, his untimely death in 1929 delayed further study.

It was not, therefore, until 1937 that Dr Conrad Elvehjem at the University of Wisconsin identified the pellagra-preventing factor as nicotinic acid. He obtained it from liver, but his studies were helped by the discovery that a similar disease in dogs known as Canine Black Tongue was also due to nicotinic acid deficiency – yet another example where a laboratory animal model was available to act as a testing system. Once this was established, clinicians soon demonstrated dramatic cures of pellagra by administering this relatively simple chemical substance, nicotinic acid.

Diet Deficient in Nicotinic Acid

The reasons why pellagra was prevalent in the southern United States and, indeed, is still widespread in other parts of the world, is a classic example of how poor diet can contribute to development of disease. We know now that nicotinic acid not only occurs in foods but can be synthesized in the body itself from another dietary constituent, the amino acid L-tryptophan. The conversion is not great, 60mg L-tryptophan is only equivalent to 1mg nicotinic acid, but it assumes importance when it represents the only source of the vitamin.

The people who developed pellagra lived on a diet consisting of maize (corn) products such as cornmeal, cornstarch, corn syrup, along with pork fat, white flour and white sugar, all of which were cheap and readily available. Maize and other cereals all contain nicotinic acid, but it is in a form that cannot be assimilated. It is significant that in Mexico, maize is also a main item in the staple diet but, in baking tortillas, Mexicans treat the flour with alkali and this releases the nicotinic acid which is then fully available. The cooking methods of the Americans did not release the vitamin, so they were denied its benefit. None of the other foods contained significant amounts of nicotinic acid and this lack, coupled with the fact that maize protein is very poor in L-tryptophan, meant that their intake of nicotinic acid was very low indeed. The incorporation of a little lean meat or dairy products into their diets would have prevented pellagra from developing.

There are two forms of the vitamin, nicotinic acid and nicotinamide. Both perform the same vitamin functions within the body and are equally effective in preventing a nutritional deficiency. Nicotinamide tends to be used when enriching foods because at high levels it has less side-effects than the acid. Where the two differ is in their therapeutic uses and these will be discussed later in the chapter.

Symptoms of Deficiency

Within the body cells, nicotinic acid, in the form of nicotinamide, is an integral part of two respiratory co-enzymes known as NAD (nicotinamide adenine dinucleotide) and NADP (nicotinamide adenine dinucleotide phosphate). These coenzymes assist in the breakdown and utilization of carbohydrates, fats and protein. They thus occupy a central role in the production of energy and in the maintenance of healthy body tissue. Nicotinic acid is effective in improving blood circulation by dilating the blood vessels and in reducing the cholesterol level of the blood. It is essential for the proper utilization of the brain and nervous system and for maintaining a healthy skin, tongue and digestive organs.

The reliance of these tissues on nicotinic acid (or nicotinamide) is reflected in what goes wrong when the vitamin is lacking. Gross deficiency leads to pellagra, characterized by the three D's, dermatitis, diarrhoea and dementia, leading eventually to the fourth, death. In the early stages of deficiency there is muscular weakness, general fatigue, anorexia, indigestion and minor skin complaints. Other non-specific symptoms include insomnia, irritability, stress and depression, all related to the nervous system. Gastro-intestinal upsets are characterized by nausea, vomiting and sometimes inflammation of the mouth and digestive tract. A feature of both mild and gross deficiency of the vitamin is a rough skin, which gave rise to the name pellagra by the Italian Physician Frapolli (1771) coined from 'pelle' meaning 'skin' and 'agra' meaning 'rough'. Hence skin lesions are the third group of symptoms associated with nicotinic acid deficiency. They include rashes on the uncovered parts of the body and dry scaly skin with wrinkles and a coarse texture.

How to Obtain Nicotinic Acid

In determining the amount of nicotinic acid in foods, there are three factors to consider: first, the level of the vitamin available; second, the level of the bound vitamin; and third, the vitamin derived from L-tryptophan. For example 77 per cent of the vitamin is in the bound form (known as niacytin) in wheat flour and how much is liberated depends upon the time of baking. Using alkaline baking powders frees all the vitamin for absorption. Fortunately, nicotinic acid is very stable to all conditions of cooking and the main losses, like those of other B vitamins, are due to leaching into water and meat drippings. Hence, as long as these liquids are consumed, you can safely assume that the vitamin in foods (apart from cereals) will usually be utilized when eaten. Rich sources of nicotinic acid include lean meats, wheatgerm, organ meats, fish and yeast extracts with some grains. Cereals provide moderate quantities of the vitamin, keeping in mind the reservations mentioned above. Instant coffee, whether decaffeinated or not, is a good source of nicotinic acid. Vegetables, green and root, are poor sources along with dairy products. Food levels are given in Table 2.

Nicotinic acid daily requirements are the highest amongst the true vitamins of the B-complex. The U.K. authorities recommend minimum amounts for adults of 18mg for men and 15mg for women, plus 3mg extra during pregnancy and 6mg extra when lactating. Growing children need from 10mg to 19mg depending upon age.

Causes of Deficiency of Nicotinic Acid

The most likely cause of low body levels of nicotinic acid is a poor diet that is low in content of the vitamin and sometimes coupled with a high intake of cereals that contain it in a non-available form. Alcoholism can also lead to nicotinic acid deficiency both through the poor diet associated with the condition and the effect of alcohol on absorption and utilization of the vitamin. The only drugs that appear to increase the need for nicotinic acid are some used in leukaemia based on 6-mercaptopurine. It is generally recommended that 50mg of the vitamin per day is sufficient to overcome the deficiencies induced by these agents, including alcohol.

Therapeutic Uses of Nicotinic Acid and Nicotinamide

Schizophrenia

The mental symptoms associated with subclinical or mild pellagra are similar to those seen in schizophrenia and include tension, depression, personality problems and mental fatigue. These observations led Drs H. Osmond and A. Hoffer of the University of Saskatchewan in Canada to suggest that this particular mental disease may respond to nicotinic acid in the same way as those who suffer from pellagra.

In February 1952 these doctors treated their first schizophrenic patients with high doses (3g to 6g) of the vitamin and reported dramatic results. They postulated that these patients had a biochemical abnormality that demanded a higher than normal intake of nicotinic acid so that even a good diet, supplying enough of the vitamin for the usual individual, was not sufficient. Dr Linus Pauling, who pioneered medical treatment with massive doses of vitamin C, suggested that a normal dietary intake of nicotinic acid could lead to a localized deficiency of the vitamin in the brain of these people. Although there was sufficient nicotinic acid to prevent the other symptoms of deficiency affecting the skin and digestive system, he believed that there was an abnormal barrier to the vitamin between the blood and brain in schizophrenia so that the latter was ostensibly starved of the vitamin.

Since these early successes, many doctors have reported similar results and clinics devoted to what is termed megavitamin therapy have been founded. One such clinic is in New York where Dr D. Hawkins has treated more than 4,000 patients with high doses of nicotinic acid. Where the acid cannot be tolerated at high levels, the neutral nicotinamide may be used. Sometimes better results were obtained when vitamin C was given at the same time. Doses of 4g each of nicotinic acid and vitamin C were required daily in some cases, with occasionally 50mg of vitamin B_6. Dr A. Cott reported in the journal Schizophrenia (1970) that it was also possible to administer high doses of these vitamins by injection in acute cases of the disease, but oral treatment could continue for several years.

No one should attempt self-treatment with these massive doses since each individual requires different amounts that depend upon personal requirements as well as upon any other treatments utilizing drugs. It must also be said there are clinical studies on record where no response was obtained when treating schizophrenics with nicotinic acid. Dr C. C. Pfieffer, Chairman of the Brain Biocentre at Princeton, New Jersey believes that schizophrenic patients who have a high level of histamine in their bodies are less likely to respond to megadose nicotinic acid, and this may explain the varying responses to megavitamin therapy.

Schizophrenic children may also respond to high doses of nicotinic acid or nicotinamide. Three grams of the vitamin, plus 500mg of vitamin B_6 daily were reported by Dr A. Hoffer to be of value in treating them and also hyperactive children. Those with poor learning ability often responded to 1-2g of nicotinic acid daily with the addition of the same amount of vitamin C, plus 200-400mg of vitamin B_6. Dr A. Cott believes that the reason for many of these mental diseases associated with childhood lies partly in an unbalanced diet high in refined foods plus an unusual demand for certain vitamins because of some biochemical abnormality. Whatever the reasons, what is certain is that many children will respond to megavitamin therapy when this is applied under medical supervision.

Alcoholism

Alcoholics often show mental symptoms similar to those of schizophrenia and are treated in a similar fashion. Daily doses of up to 6g per day of either nicotinic acid or nicotinamide were given to more than 500 alcoholics over a period of 18 months in a study run by Dr R. F. Smith of Michigan. Only 66 patients showed a response classified as poor, with all others varying from fair up to excellent. What was particularly encouraging was that not only did mental symptoms improve, but that many of the individuals were actually cured of the alcohol habit. The response to the vitamin was superior to many standard drug treatments. Nicotinic acid can also help some tobacco addicts stop the habit, not surprisingly perhaps since both smoking and drinking introduce the same poison, acetaldehyde, into the body system.

Reducing the Blood Cholesterol

Nicotinic acid, but not nicotinamide, will reduce cholesterol levels in the blood. In a short term trial at the Mayo Clinic in 1956, 3g of nicotinic acid were given orally to patients with high blood cholesterol and levels were lowered to normal in 72 per cent of those tested. The remaining 28 per cent responded favourably to 4-6g per day. A longer term study over 11 years was carried out at the Dartmouth-Hitchcock Medical Centre in New Hampshire. A dose of 100mg nicotinic acid was given to 160 patients after each meal and this was increased over 11 days to 1g after each meal, at which level therapy continued. The average decrease in plasma cholesterol was 26 per cent in those who took the vitamin for at least one year, and the lower cholesterol level was maintained for as long as treatment continued. It was particularly gratifying to note that there were no serious side-effects.

Other studies in Britain have indicated that nicotinic acid also has the property of lowering blood fats (triglycerides) in general at the above doses. In this respect it appears to be as effective as the drug clofibrate. It is believed to act in two ways: first, by inhibiting the synthesis of fats in the blood; and second, by competing with and preventing the release of free fatty acids which combine with cholesterol.

Use in Arthritis

As long ago as 1941, nicotinic acid was found to relieve the symptoms of arthritis and other joint malfunctions. Dr W. Kaufman reported that his patients, treated with large doses of the vitamin, found their joint mobility increased, stiffness and deformity of the joint decreased and pain was relieved. Further studies from the same source on a total of 663 patients showed that those on 3 to 6g per day actually gained in muscle strength, experienced decreased fatigue and were relieved of the chronic emotional disorders associated with the disease. Dr A. Hoffer, the pioneer of megavitamin therapy in schizophrenia, confirmed the beneficial effects of either nicotinic acid or nicotinamide in his arthritic patients in the *Canadian Medical Association Journal* (1959). He stressed that although relief is often immediate, long term benefits can only come with prolonged therapy.

Toxic Effects of Nicotinic Acid and Nicotinamide

Nicotinic acid causes blood vessels to dilate and so, when given in large doses, it may cause flushing of the face, a sensation of heat and a pounding headache. These symptoms are of a transient nature but can be distressing to some. None of these effects are associated with nicotinamide. This action on the minor blood vessels explains how it is of benefit in relieving chilblains (induced by contraction of blood vessels) but a better response is obtained if vitamin K is taken at the same time. Due to its dilating properties, nicotinic acid was banned some years ago as a food preservative. Susceptible individuals often showed ill-effects because of the high levels of the nicotinic acid added to tinned meats. Nicotinamide is not without its side-effects and in large doses may cause depression in some adults. Liver malfunction may also result from this form of the vitamin, although doses above 3g per day are needed before symptoms appear. According to Drs M. M. Nelson and J. O. Forfar writing in the *British Medical Journal* (1971), high doses of nicotinamide should be avoided during pregnancy, particularly during the first 56 days, to prevent possible malformations of the foetus.

Other toxic symptoms reported with high doses of nicotinic acid include dry skin, rashes, itching and boils. Abdominal cramps, diarrhoea and nausea sometimes appear. An increase in blood uric acid leading to mild gout symptoms occasionally result from 6g of nicotinic acid taken on a regular basis. All these symptoms disappear when treatment with the vitamin ceases. Such high doses of nicotinic acid should not be taken by anyone suffering from gastric or duodenal ulcers since the vitamin in this form can irritate the ulcer. The record for excessive intake of nicotinic acid must belong to a patient of Dr A. Hoffer. He took 90g in a suicide attempt, but the only result was nausea, vomiting and diarrhoea.

2

THE ANTI-DEPRESSION VITAMIN

During studies on experimental rats at the University of Pennsylvania in 1934 it was noted that on certain diets the animals developed a dermatitis that did not respond to any of the known vitamins. Professor Paul Gyorgy at the Department of Medicine then isolated a factor from liver that cured the disease and the new vitamin was designated B_6, later given the name 'pyridoxine'.

In food the vitamin exists in three forms known as pyridoxine, pyridoxal, and pyridoxamine. All three are equally acceptable to the human body as vitamins and are converted after absorption into the biologically-active form known as pyridoxal-5-phosphate. As this compound, vitamin B_6 is involved in more than sixty enzymic reactions and is essential for sustaining life. Many of these are concerned with the metabolism of the amino acids supplied by the protein we eat, either by making certain amino acids from others or by reactions that convert some amino acids to substances that are essential for nerve and brain function. Hence, lack of the vitamin can give rise to nervous problems, mental depression, and convulsions, particularly in infants.

Other signs of deficiency include skin complaints, sore tongue and a particular type of anaemia that is cured only by vitamin B_6.

All three forms of vitamin B_6 appear to be stable to most cooking methods. None are affected by acids, alkalis or oxidation, so losses tend to be due to leaching out into cooking water. Considerable destruction of the vitamin can occur in milk that has been treated at high temperature, probably because of its interaction with other components of milk. When such milk was fed to babies they often suffered from convulsions due solely to the lack of vitamin B_6. Once this was realized, modern methods of drying milk were developed that did not cause the wholesale destruction of the vitamin and so the problem was overcome.

Sources of Vitamin B_6

Vitamin B_6 is widely distributed in foods of all kinds and is particularly rich in liver, kidney, pork, ham and veal amongst the meats; fresh fish; bananas, avocados, prunes, raisins; peanuts, walnuts and wholegrain cereals. Its occurrence in various foods is given in Table 3.

There are three amino acids which, as well as being converted into body protein, also undergo other reactions to give compounds that have a direct bearing on the functioning of the brain and nervous system and probably also on the blood circulation. They are known as L-tryptophan, L-glutamic acid and L-methionine. Now that we know that the metabolism of these three essential amino acids is under the direct control of, and is absolutely dependent on, vitamin B_6, the manifestations of its deficiency become apparent.

Detecting B_6 Deficiency

How do we know that vitamin B_6 is deficient in an individual? The simplest method is the tryptophan loading test. In this the person is given between 2g and 5g of L-tryptophan dissolved in a drink. If they are deficient in vitamin B_6 certain compounds are excreted in the urine in

Table 3.
The Vitamin B_6 Content of Raw Foods (mg per 100g)

Food Item	Pyridoxine (Vitamin B_6)
Liver (pig)	0.68
Kidney (pig)	0.25
Beef	0.32
Lamb	0.25
Pork	0.45
Chicken	0.42
Fish (white)	0.33
Fish (fatty)	0.45
Eggs (whole)	0.11
Milk (cows)	0.04
Cheese (hard)	0.08
Cheese (cottage)	0.01
Yogurt	0.04
Wholemeal bread	0.14
White bread	0.08
Wheat bran	1.38
Wheatgerm	0.92
Wheat grains	0.50
Oatflakes	0.75
Maize (corn)	0.06
Rice (unpolished, brown)	0.42
Soya flour (full fat)	0.57
Citrus fruits (peeled)	0.06
Dried fruits	0.10
Bananas	0.51
Nuts (fresh)	0.50
Nuts (roasted)	0.40
Potatoes	0.25
Root vegetables (carrots etc.)	0.15
Greenleaf vegetables	0.16
Pulses (beans, peas etc.)	0.16
Yeast (brewer's, dried)	4.2
Yeast extract	1.3

large amounts and these can be measured. They are partially-converted L-tryptophan and they accumulate because lack of B_6 means they cannot be converted any further. They have the tongue-twisting names of xan-thurenic acid, 3-hydroxykynurenine and kynurenine. An excessive excretion of these compounds in the urine indicate a vitamin B_6 deficiency. Once the individual is treated with the vitamin, the levels of these compounds drop in the urine, indicating that the B_6 is once again taking over its proper functions.

L-tryptophan is converted into two very important substances within the body and both mechanisms are under the control of vitamin B_6. One set of reactions produces the other B vitamin nicotinic acid, and this was discussed in Chapter 1. The second series of reactions produces a compound called serotonin which is essential for brain and nerve function. In the absence of vitamin B_6, both mech-anisms fail and it is lack of serotonin formation that is a factor in inducing depression.

Vitamin B_6 and Depression

Production of serotonin takes place constantly in the brain and at nerve endings. When it does not, serotonin levels drop and the results are a form of depression and sleep disturbances. This is because the control of mood is dependent on brain concentrations of serotonin. Anything that interferes with production of serotonin must, therefore, be reflected in mental attitudes, so perhaps it is not surprising that a vitamin B_6 deficiency first manifests itself as a mental condition.

In various studies, between 75 per cent and 100 per cent of women on the contraceptive pill showed abnormal metabolism of L-tryptophan indicated by the tryptophan loading test. Similarly, up to 60 per cent of pregnant women showed identical findings. The factor responsible for inducing these abnormalities is believed to be the female hormone oestrogen. In the 'Pill' the oestrogen is synthetic; in pregnancy it is natural, but the effect is the same because in both cases concentrations in the blood are high. Oestrogens divert L-tryptophan from the serotonin and nicotinic acid pathways, probably by interfering with the mechanism of vitamin B_6 control. It is highly significant that many women who develop depression while using the contraceptive pill are cured by simple supplementation with vitamin B_6. In one trial carried out at St Mary's Hospital, London, a group of 39 women had depression related to taking the 'Pill'. Of these, 19 were found to have an absolute deficiency of vitamin B_6. The administration of 40mg of the vitamin per day removed the depression symptoms in all women who were B_6 deficient. No improvement was detected in the others even on prolonged B_6 treatment. Hence, in these cases the depressive state was apparently not related to B_6 deficiency, but the results do suggest that supplementation with the vitamin is a useful first line of treatment, particularly with self-medication.

Other Effects of Vitamin B_6 Deficiency

There are two side-effects of the contraceptive pill, both of which are related to the apparent vitamin B_6 deficiency induced by the hormonal constituents. The first of these involves glucose metabolism. Xanthurenic acid was mentioned as one compound that is formed in excess when there is a lack of vitamin B_6. This compound can react with the hormone insulin and inactivate it. Hence, when there is too much xanthurenic acid present in the blood, the insulin present cannot function in controlling the blood sugar levels. The result is mild diabetes that is an occasional feature noted in pregnancy and in those taking the contraceptive pill. Supplementation with the vitamin restores blood glucose levels to normal in both circumstances.

Anaemia can also be induced by lack of vitamin B_6. The active form of the vitamin known as pyridoxal-5-phosphate is known to be essential in the production of haemoglobin, the red pigment in blood that carries oxygen. Taking the 'Pill' for any length of time may slow down the production of haemoglobin resulting in an anaemia that responds only to vitamin B_6. Treatment with any other anti-anaemia preparations like iron, copper, folic acid and vitamin B_{12} gives no response.

Vitamin B_6 and the Premenstrual Syndrome (PMS)

The main premenstrual syndrome symptoms are depression, irritability, tiredness, breast discomfort, swollen abdomen and puffy fingers and ankles. The similarity of the depression of PMS with that suffered by the 'Pill'-users led research workers at St Thomas's Hospital PMS Clinic to assess treatment of the condition with simple supplementation of vitamin B_6. The results were very exciting. When given in doses of 100mg per day, from day 10 of one cycle to day 3 of the next, the vitamin caused an overall improvement in all symptoms in 63 per cent of the patients. This was extremely favourable when compared to the improvement in 73 per cent of the patients treated with conventional hormones. One significant difference was the complete lack of side-effects in the vitamin-treated females, unlike those treated with hormones. Although the results are preliminary, vitamin B_6 supplementation would appear to be a simple first-line treatment of PMS, especially as over 80 per cent of the women tested were cured of premenstrual headache, the most common symptom noted.

Vitamin B_6 and Convulsions

L-glutamic acid is another essential amino acid that is converted under the influence of vitamin B_6 into a compound essential for brain function. This is known as gamma-aminobutyric acid (GABA) and is regarded as a natural calming agent produced by the central nervous system. Deficiency of vitamin B_6 may therefore cause convulsions because the brain is unable to form the compound in adequate amounts. Convulsions in infants can sometimes be related to lack of vitamin B_6 and supplementation at high doses (100mg per day upwards) can bring the convulsions under control. In these cases the deficiency is due to a genetic defect rather than a dietary deficiency of the vitamin, and is responsive only to large doses of B_6.

Vitamin B_6 and Heart Disease

The third specific amino acid that depends upon vitamin B_6 for its metabolism in the body is L-methionine. This material is converted to homocysteine which is a toxic compound. Under normal circumstances this does not matter because it, in turn, is converted very quickly into cystathionine, a very important amino acid needed for other body actions. The change from homocysteine to cystathionine is dependent upon vitamin B_6. Some unfortunate individuals are born with a hereditary defect that means they are unable to make this change, with the result that they are mentally retarded and rarely live beyond their teens. However, it is very interesting that these young people have extensive disease of the blood vessels which are thickened by the deposition of fatty plaques – a condition known as atherosclerosis. It looked as though the build-up of excessive homocysteine had prematurely given rise to this disease which is usually reserved for middle and old age.

These findings led Dr Kilner McCully working at Harvard University and the Massachusetts General Hospital to suggest in 1969 that high concentrations of homocysteine induced by a deficiency of vitamin B_6 may help to cause atherosclerosis. This conclusion was based not only on his own findings, but also on research carried out elsewhere. For example, Drs James Rinehart and Louis Greenberg of the University of California Medical School fed monkeys a diet deficient in vitamin B_6. The animals developed atherosclerosis. No other B vitamin deficiency induced the condition. Other observations include: first, when human beings and animals develop vitamin B_6 deficiency, the level of the toxic homocysteine in the blood rises; second, worldwide studies indicate that those suffering from atherosclerosis invariably have low vitamin B_6 levels in their blood; and third, those people with atherosclerosis have high levels of homocysteine in their blood. There may also be a relationship between the B_6 deficiency known to be induced by the 'Pill' and the increased occurrence of heart and blood vessel disease known to exist in those women taking this form of contraception. An English study on 46,000 women who had taken the 'Pill' for at least five years indicated that they had an incidence of heart and blood vessel disease some ten times greater than that associated with a similar number of women who practised other forms of contraception. The evidence is suggestive, but not conclusive, since their vitamin B_6 status was not measured.

It is tempting, then, to suggest that atherosclerosis is another disease related to vitamin B_6 deficiency, particularly when this may occur throughout a lifetime of bad dietary habits. Whilst the academics work out the mechanisms however, it is perhaps safer to simply ensure against even a mild deficiency of vitamin B_6 by eating the right foods, and taking supplements where food alone cannot guarantee an adequate intake as in those taking the 'Pill'.

Vitamin B_6 and Bronchial Asthma

Vitamin B_6 has been referred to as the anti-allergy vitamin, mainly on account of its successful use in some allergic skin diseases, in hay fever and in bronchial asthma. Comprehensive studies by a team of doctors at Nassau County Medical Centre, U.S.A., headed by Dr P. J. Collipp have indicated that pyridoxine is a remarkably safe and effective treatment for some asthma sufferers. The clue to the treatment was provided by the observation that many asthma victims showed abnormal metabolism of vitamin B_6 when tested with the tryptophan loading test. Consequently, in one trial, 88 asthmatic children received 100mg of vitamin B_6 twice per day and a similar number received a harmless placebo. Neither patients nor doctors knew what they were given – in fact this was a true double blind study. The effect of the treatment was assessed by noting such criteria as wheezing, difficult breathing, cough, tightness in the chest and outright asthmatic attacks.

Only starting with the second month did those receiving

vitamin B_6 show any definite clinical improvement over those receiving placebo. From then on, however, the improvement was maintained in every aspect of the disease. No side-effects were observed during the five-month duration of the trial. It must be stressed that existing drug treatment of the individuals continued, but as this was palliative rather than curative (e.g. the use of bronchodilators), it was gradually phased out under medical guidance. The researchers could not explain why the vitamin has this beneficial effect, but they admit that pyridoxine appears to be acting as a drug rather than as a vitamin. It is possible that these children are suffering from a B_6-dependency so that for some reason their requirements for the vitamin are particularly high and cannot be obtained simply from the diet. Adult sufferers from asthma also benefit from a similar dosage but the positive response to the vitamin is not as outstanding as that in children.

Vitamin B_6 and Kidney Stones
The most common kind of kidney stones are formed from an insoluble mineral called calcium oxalate. This is composed of calcium and oxalic acid, both normal constituents of food. In addition, oxalic acid is produced by the body during its normal metabolic processes. Yet some people form stones and others do not, despite having similar diets. The ability to form stones depends upon two factors: first, how well the calcium oxalate can be kept in solution; and second, the control of oxalic acid production. The first factor depends upon the presence of adequate magnesium, since the ratio of calcium to magnesium determines the solubility of calcium oxalate. The second factor is related to vitamin B_6, since when this is deficient there is an increase in oxalic acid production. Adequate pyridoxine protects by reducing the formation of this potential precipitating agent.

These observations were put to the test in a clinical study carried out at Harvard University by Drs E. L. Prienard and S. N. Gershoff and reported in the *American Journal of Clinical Nutrition* (1967). A total of 265 patients with histories of chronic kidney stone formation were treated with 240mg magnesium and 20mg of vitamin B_6 per day. A staggering 89 per cent of these patients benefited from the course of supplementation. They stopped producing kidney stones and remained free of them while on the mineral/vitamin treatment. This simple treatment is safe and effective, but it is preferably taken in conjunction with a calcium-controlled diet, a regime that many kidney stone sufferers are already familiar with.

How Safe is Vitamin B_6?

Vitamin B_6 is remarkably non-toxic. In none of the clinical trials, where doses up to 200mg daily were used, was there any report of side-effects. The only case where the vitamin may have a deleterious effect is on those patients suffering from Parkinson's disease who are being treated with levo-dopa. This is because the vitamin reduces the effects of the drug. Vitamin B_6 supplements should therefore not be taken by these people.

3

THE ANTI-STRESS VITAMINS: PANTOTHENIC ACID AND BIOTIN

The name pantothenic acid is derived from the Greek word 'panthos' which means 'everywhere', an apt name for a vitamin that is universally distributed in foods and in all living matter. After the discovery of riboflavin, nicotinic acid and pyridoxine, it was soon established that these vitamins alone were not sufficient to prevent some specific conditions in animals. For example, the new factor prevented the development of a certain type of dermatitis found only around the eyes and beaks of chicks. It also had the ability to prevent the greying of hair in black rats. Fortunately, an identical factor was also needed for growth of yeast, so a simple test system for the factor utilizing this micro-organism was soon developed. The assay enabled Dr R. J. Williams of the University of Texas to isolate the new vitamin from rice husks in 1939.

The Function of Pantothenic Acid
The universal distribution of pantothenic acid in plant and animal cells reflects its profound importance. It functions as a constituent of coenzyme A which is essential for energy

production, for fat and cholesterol metabolism, for antibody formation and to ensure a healthy nervous system. Its involvement with cholesterol is particularly important since this compound is the starting material for production of anti-stress hormones by the body. Pantothenic acid is necessary to convert cholesterol into these essential components.

No specific deficiency symptoms in man have been associated with pantothenic acid apart perhaps from the 'burning feet' syndrome. The earliest symptoms are aching, burning or throbbing in the feet. These discomforts become more intense and develop into sharp, stabbing, shooting pains that may spread as far as the knee causing agonizing pain. The disease is associated with poor diet and responds to pantothenic acid treatment. It is by no means certain that pantothenic acid is the only vitamin deficient and the condition may be due to a generalized deficiency. Studies on human volunteers have indicated that signs of pantothenic acid deficiency, such as loss of appetite, indigestion, abdominal pain, respiratory infections, neuritis, arm and leg cramps and lack of hormone production, may be associated with lack of other vitamins as well as pantothenic acid. Mental symptoms also accompany the deficiency, including insomnia, fatigue and depression. Alcoholics are particularly prone to nervous disease and psychosis that may be related to pantothenic acid deficiency.

Dietary Loss of Pantothenic Acid
What are the chances of becoming deficient in pantothenic acid? The answer, like that of so many of the B-complex members, lies in the quality of the diet and how it is cooked. Although the vitamin is widely distributed, substantial losses can occur during the dry-processing of foods. Production of white flour from wholegrain wheat results in wholesale destruction and loss. Domestic cooking processes and baking cause little loss of the vitamin apart from roasting of meat which can destroy 40 per cent of the content. It is water-soluble, so losses into cooking water and

the thawed drippings from frozen meat can be considerable. Acid and alkaline conditions during cooking are particularly destructive to pantothenic acid, so such aids as vinegar and sodium bicarbonate, for example, should be avoided during cooking procedures.

Requirements

The human requirements for pantothenic acid are thought to be about 10mg per day, but this should be considered an absolute minimum in view of the evidence (presented later) that low intakes of the vitamin may be related to degenerative diseases. There is an increased requirement for the vitamin during any sort of stress situation, after an injury and following antibiotic therapy. It is necessary in the latter case because intestinal bacteria synthesize the vitamin and so provide an important source. Hence, any prolonged anti-biotic treatment may destroy the 'friendly' bacteria that normally inhabit the gut and one of the sources of panto-thenic acid is lost. The side-effects and toxicity associated with the antibiotics streptomycin, neomycin, kanamycin and viomycin are also lessened with pantothenic acid supplements, but the reasons are not known.

The largest quantities of pantothenic acid are found in meat, poultry, fish, wholegrain cereals and legumes. Fruit, vegetables and milk represent other less rich sources. Levels of pantothenic acid in foods are given in Table 4.

The vitamin pantothenic acid is a pale-yellow, oily liquid that is unstable in the pure state. For this reason it is incorporated into such dietary supplements as calcium pantothenate, a crystalline powder that is far more stable. Calcium pantothenate is just as effective a vitamin as the naturally occurring pantothenic acid itself. For the same reasons you may see the vitamin offered as dexpanthenol or pantothenol, a simple derivative that is readily converted by the body to pantothenic acid. In this form it is incorporated into creams, ointments, shampoos and other cosmetic products.

Table 4.
The Pantothenic Acid and Biotin Content of Raw Foods

Food Item	Pantothenic Acid (mg per 100g)	Biotin (mcg per 100g)
Liver (pig)	6.5	27
Kidney (pig)	3.0	32
Beef	0.7	3
Lamb	0.7	2
Pork	1.1	3
Chicken	1.2	2
Fish (white)	0.2	3
Fish (fatty)	2.0	5
Eggs (whole)	1.8	25
Milk (cows)	0.35	2
Cheese (hard)	0.3	2
Cheese (cottage)	0.4	2
Yogurt	0.4	2
Wholemeal bread	0.6	6
White bread	0.3	1
Wheat bran	2.4	14
Wheatgerm	2.2	12
Wheatgrains	0.8	7
Oatflakes	0.9	20
Maize (corn)	0.6	6
Rice (unpolished, brown)	0.6	3
Soya flour (full fat)	1.8	–
Citrus fruits (peeled)	0.25	1
Dried fruits	0.70	–
Bananas	0.26	–
Nuts (fresh)	2.7	–
Nuts (roasted)	2.1	–
Potatoes	0.30	0.1
Root vegetables (carrots etc.)	0.25	0.6
Greenleaf vegetables	0.21	0.1
Pulses (beans, peas etc.)	0.75	0.5
Yeast (brewer's, dried)	9.5	80
Yeast extract	3.8	27

Pantothenic Acid and Resistance to Infection

One of the commoner features of pantothenic acid deficiency in man and experimental animals is their lowered resistance to attack by infectious bacteria and viruses. Experimental studies carried out, in 1971 by Dr A. E. Axelrod of the Pittsburgh University Medical School, on mice subjected to bacterial attack, indicated that pantothenic acid deficiency laid the animals wide open to respiratory infection. A similar lack of resistance was a feature of human volunteers from whom pantothenic acid was witheld. The reason is that this vitamin, along with vitamin B_6, appears to be essential in the production of antibodies, those factors produced by the body to help neutralize the invading bacteria and viruses. Such attack by harmful micro-organisms represents a stress upon the body itself and here pantothenic acid is fulfilling one of its roles as an anti-stress agent.

Pantothenic Acid and Allergy

An allergy may be defined as a sensitivity or over-reaction of the body to foreign substances via the stomach, via the respiratory tract or upon the skin. Like microbial infections, they stimulate the body to give a response and hence exert stress reaction. Lack of pantothenic acid will intensify an allergic response in both animals and man. For example, it was reported in *Acta Paediatrica* (1963) by Dr I. Szorady at the University Medical School in Szegad, Hungary, that giving pantothenic acid (100mg orally) to children resulted in a decrease of allergic skin reactions by as much as 50 per cent. Dr Sandra M. Stewart, a paediatrician from Columbus, Ohio, herself suffered from an allergy problem, but in her case the respiratory system was affected. Simply taking 100mg of pantothenic acid at night prevented the excess mucous secretion which was giving rise in the morning to cough and the stuffed-up feeling associated with the allergy. No one is quite sure how pantothenic acid may help in reducing the allergic response, but it could be via the same mechanisms that cause the body to defeat invading micro-organisms – both very much dependent on adequate supplies of the vitamin.

Pantothenic Acid and Arthritis

The first clue that there may be a connection between pantothenic acid and arthritis came with the observation that young rats deprived of the vitamin developed joint inflammation and the hardening of their bones was impaired. This supported previous studies that showed that pigs and dogs developed arthritic symptoms akin to those in human beings when pantothenic acid was missing from their diets. A significant report then appeared in *The Lancet* (1963) regarding the blood pantothenic acid levels of various groups of people, with and without arthritis. What emerged was that vegetarians had significantly higher blood levels of pantothenic acid than those on a meat-eating diet. The common factor in those suffering from arthritis, whether they were vegetarian or not, was the greatly reduced levels of pantothenic acid in their blood. In fact, the lower the level of pantothenic acid in the blood, the more severe were the symptoms of arthritis.

The two authors, Drs E. C. Barton-Wright and W. A. Elliott then proceeded to test their hypothesis that rheumatoid arthritis is a vitamin-deficiency disease by treating arthritic patients with daily injections of 50mg calcium pantothenate. Within seven days, the blood levels of the vitamin increased and this was paralleled by alleviation of the arthritic symptoms. This improvement stayed at this level despite further treatment for three weeks. However, discontinuing the supplementary calcium pantothenate caused the symptoms to return. Another report in the same journal from Dr J. C. Annand claimed a similar result with the more serious disorder of osteo-arthritis.

These encouraging results led to a much larger trial of the vitamin in arthritis organized by the General Practitioner Research Group and reported in *The Practitioner* (1980). A total of 94 patients were involved and neither they nor the doctors knew whether the treatment was calcium pantothenate or a harmless placebo. Response to the treatment was assessed both by doctor and patient using a number of criteria. The dosage regime used was 500mg (1 tablet) daily for 2 days, 1000mg (2 tablets) for 3 days, 1500mg (3 tablets) for 4 days and finally 2000mg (4 tablets) per day thereafter for a period of 2 months. Highly significant effects were recorded for calcium pantothenate in reducing the duration of morning stiffness, the degree of disability and the severity of pain.

Only in the condition of rheumatoid arthritis, however, was there any indication of a beneficial effect – there was little if any in the other types of arthritis. Why pantothenic acid should have this beneficial effect is not known with certainty, but an important clue lies in its function in controlling the synthesis of the anti-stress hormones of the body. Lack of the vitamin means lowered production of these hormones with subsequent development of inflammatory and degenerative diseases like arthritis. The ultimate treatment for these diseases consists of highly potent synthetic hormones known as corticosteroids. Pantothenic acid may enable the glands of the body to produce its own natural corticosteroids, so the end effect of either treatment is probably the same, but the vitamin therapy of course is far safer.

Although pantothenic acid treatment of arthritis is encouraging, it is treating a pre-existing condition. Perhaps the condition would not arise at all if we all had a truly adequate intake of pantothenic acid from birth. 50mg per day should be regarded as a minimum meaningful dose that we should obtain from our food supplements. At least there is no evidence that calcium pantothenate is toxic, even in quantities far in excess of this.

Biotin
Like so many of the B vitamins, the discovery of biotin was a combination of chance and astute observation. It had been noted that when rats were fed raw egg white as a sole source of protein, they developed dermatitis and blood disorders. In addition, they suffered widespread hair-loss, their limbs became paralysed, and there was drastic weight-loss leading eventually to death. These symptoms were associated only

with raw egg white – cooking the egg white first kept the animals healthy. Supplementation with other foods prevented the symptoms from developing, even in the presence of raw egg white. It was assumed that egg white as the sole source of protein in a diet caused a deficiency in an important dietary factor, and Dr Paul Gyorgy eventually isolated this factor from liver during the early 1940s. It was given the name 'biotin' when it was found to be identical to a micro-organism growth factor known as 'bios'.

Deficiency in Man

The reason why raw egg white induces a biotin deficiency is that this food contains a protein, avidin, which binds biotin and prevents its absorption from the intestine. Cooking egg white denatures avidin so that it can no longer bind the vitamin which then becomes available to the body. It is therefore possible to produce biotin deficiency in man by feeding dried egg white as the sole source of protein. When this was done with human volunteers the subjects developed symptoms associated with biotin deficiency after ten weeks on the diet. They were fatigued, depressed and sleepy with nausea and loss of appetite. Muscular pains developed and they lost their reflexes. The tongue became pale and smooth. Skin diseases appeared that would not respond to other vitamins. The blood level of cholesterol increased and a particular type of anaemia became evident. All of these symptoms disappeared with injections of 150 to 300 micrograms of biotin daily.

Outright biotin deficiency is rare in man, but when it occurs it is always associated with unusual diets. In 1943 it was reported in the *New England Journal of Medicine* that an eccentric who lived on six dozen raw eggs weekly washed down with four quarts of red wine developed a severe dermatitis that was only relieved with biotin injections. A boy who was suffering from an illness that necessitated a diet of six raw eggs per day delivered by gastric tube was reported in 1968 as developing scaly dermatitis with loss of hair. Both conditions responded only to biotin. There are other cases on record and the common symptoms appear to be dermatitis and hair loss.

Some babies develop seborrhoeic dermatitis (dry scaling of the scalp and face) with persistent diarrhoea soon after birth and the reason can be traced to a lack of biotin. Human milk has a particularly low content of biotin and the small quantity present is bound to protein. If the infant does not have the capacity to digest this protein efficiently, the biotin is not available to him. Treatment is therefore by injection of the vitamin. At the same time the nursing mother is fed biotin-rich foods like liver to boost the concentration of the vitamin in her milk.

Functions of Biotin

Biotin is now known to be a coenzyme for a wide variety of body functions. It is required for the metabolism of carbohydrates, proteins and fats both in their involvement in production of energy and in their conversion to important substances. Biotin is necessary in the metabolism of the essential polyunsaturated acids and its deficiency effects upon the skin and hair may relate directly to this function. In babies for example, reports in *The Lancet* of 1979 and 1980 indicate that seborrhoeic dermatitis can sometimes be helped by linoleic acid (a polyunsaturated fatty acid), although the results are not as dramatic as those obtained with biotin. Hence the vitamin is needed for growth and the maintenance of healthy skin, hair, sweat glands, nerves, bone marrow and the glands producing sex hormones. Malfunction of these roles explain the various manifestations of biotin deficiency.

Sources of Biotin

Biotin accompanies the rest of the B-complex vitamins in such varied foods as yeast, liver, eggs, wholegrains, nuts and fish (see Table 4, page 49).

Losses occur during cooking processes mainly due to a leaching out into cooking water. The drying of milk for baby foods used to cause serious losses of the vitamin but the vitamin can now be synthesized and so such milks are now supplemented.

It is likely that most of the biotin that man requires is obtained not from the food, but by intestinal bacterial synthesis. The quantity excreted is often more than that taken in the diet, suggesting that this is an important source. Hence any antibiotic that can destroy the intestinal bacterial population may contribute to reduced intakes of the vitamin. Sulphonamides are particularly active in this respect since they are often not absorbed and survive down the gastro-intestinal tract. Supplementation with biotin is sensible during prolonged antibiotic therapy.

Therapeutic Use

Apart from a trial of supplementary biotin in skin complaints, alopecia and other scalp conditions, there is little else likely to respond to high doses of the vitamin. However, recently research has indicated a possible relationship between biotin and sudden infant death syndrome or cot deaths. An Australian group were researching unexpected deaths in young chickens and found that the birds were lacking in biotin and had apparently succumbed to mild stress exposure. Upon learning of this work and realizing the similarities, a U.K. group researching cot deaths at Sheffield Children's Hospital, used similar techniques to determine the biotin levels in the liver of the babies who had died. Sure enough, these infants all had deficiency of biotin. Similarly all the babies at Sheffield were known to have suffered from some mild complaint that was not fatal in itself but was capable of inducing a mild stress reaction.

Why should babies be deficient in biotin? It is probably because at birth infants have no intestinal bacteria so this source of biotin is denied them. We have seen previously that milk is not a very good source of the vitamin, so the levels in their food could be low. This combination of factors can thus lead to a deficiency of biotin.

It is not suggested that biotin deficiency itself is the cause of death but, in the words of the researchers, 'it may leave the infant in a condition in which cot death can be triggered by mild stress, for example, infection, a missed meal, excessive heat or cold, or a changed environment'.

Daily intakes of biotin have been put at between 150 and 300mcg, but this is difficult to assess in view of the intestinal synthesis of the vitamin. No toxic effects at supplementation levels above this (e.g. 10mg per day in infants) have ever been reported.

4
THE ANTI-ANAEMIA VITAMINS: FOLIC ACID AND VITAMIN B$_{12}$

The first clue that lack of dietary factors could produce a specific type of anaemia was provided by the studies of Dr Lucy Wills (1931) in India. Pregnant women were prone to a particular type of anaemia that did not respond to any of the known vitamins nor to liver extract, but was cured by an autolysed yeast preparation. Liver extract was known to help in cases of pernicious anaemia, so it was obvious that the anaemia of pregnancy was of a different type.

The diet of these women was mainly composed of polished rice and white bread and was obviously deficient in some essential component. Then occurred one of those happy chances, so prevalent in the early days of vitamin research, when completely unrelated investigations by a group of American biochemists in 1941 revealed that a factor in spinach cured a dietary anaemia in chicks. In 1945 the material became available in larger quantities and Dr Tom Spies demonstrated that the compound, named 'folic acid', because of its occurrence in green foliage, cured the anaemia of pregnancy, described by Dr Lucy Wills some 15 years earlier.

Oddly enough, the importance of folic acid had been predicted from studies carried out in 1885 by Dr Gowland Hopkins when he described the colour pigments of butter-flies' wings. These are related chemically to folic acid although no one has yet suggested these beautiful objects as a source of the vitamin!

Occurrence of Folic Acid

Folic acid occurs in many different guises in food and in body tissues and not all of them are utilized as a vitamin. For example, in food between 30 and 75 per cent of the folic acid present occurs as conjugated forms that are converted to the vitamin by the digestive processes. The remainder of the folic acid cannot be utilized by animal tissues and so has no vitamin activity. Folic acid is widely distributed throughout foods, but there is vast variation in the quantity present. The richest sources are liver, oysters and yeast extracts, but green vegetables yield meaningful amounts of the vitamin. These foodstuffs also contain the highest proportion of available folate (salt of folic acid). Milk, fruits and most meats yield little of the vitamin. Table 5 summarizes the folic acid content of various foods.

Cooking of foods in large volumes of water causes leaching out of the folic acid content, so the rule is to boil vegetables in the smallest amount of water possible. Oxygen accelerates the breakdown of the vitamin at high temper-atures and the simplest natural protective agent is vitamin C. In the presence of this vitamin, folic acid is much more stable, so it is fortuitous that both tend to occur together in green vegetables although, in view of the instability of vitamin C in foodstuffs, the amount of the naturally occurring compound may not be sufficient. Folic acid is also unstable to light especially in the presence of riboflavin (vitamin B_2). Overall losses of 45 per cent of the total folic acid can occur in processing and cooking of vegetables, fruits and dairy products, so the rule would appear to be, eat these foods fresh and raw.

Table 5.
Folic Acid and Vitamin B₁₂ Content of Raw Foods

Food Item	Folic Acid (mcg per 100g)	Vitamin B₁₂ (mcg per 100g)
Liver (pig)	110	25
Kidney (pig)	42	14
Beef	10	2
Lamb	5	2
Pork	5	3
Chicken	12	0.5
Fish (white)	12	2
Fish (fatty)	26	5
Eggs (whole)	30	2
Milk (cows)	5	0.3
Cheese (hard)	20	1.5
Cheese (cottage)	9	0.5
Yogurt	2	0.1
Wholemeal bread	39	0
White bread	27	0
Wheat bran	260	0
Wheatgerm	310	0
Wheatgrains	57	0
Oatflakes	60	0
Maize (corn)	10	0
Rice (unpolished, brown)	29	0
Soya flour (full fat)	430	0
Citrus fruits (peeled)	37	0
Dried fruits	14	0
Bananas	22	0
Nuts (fresh)	110	0
Nuts (roasted)	57	0
Potatoes	14	0
Root vegetables (carrots etc.)	15	0
Greenleaf vegetables	90	0
Pulses (beans, peas etc.)	80	0
Yeast (brewer's, dried)	2400	0

Daily Requirements

According to a study reported in the *American Journal of Clinical Nutrition* (1973), a mixed Western type diet will provide 150 to 300 micrograms of folic acid in its various forms daily. The U.K. authorities (D.H.S.S. Report 15, 1979) recommend 300 micrograms per day for all adults apart from pregnant and lactating women who need 500 and 400 micrograms respectively. These figures suggest that much of the population must be on the borderline of folic acid deficiency. Vegetarians, however, have less need to worry because their high intake of green leaf vegetables will supply ample folic acid.

Symptoms of Folic Acid Deficiency

Lack of folic acid gives rise to megaloblastic anaemia. In this condition the red blood cells become very large and uneven in size and shape and they have a much shorter life-span than normal red blood cells. The outward signs of deficiency are similar to those associated with other types of anaemia. These include weakness, fatigue, irritability, sleeplessness, culminating in mild mental symptoms such as forgetfulness and confusion.

Function of Folic Acid in the Body

Folic acid is essential in the metabolism of the nucleic acids which are of two types: ribonucleic acids (RNA) and deoxyribonucleic acids (DNA). These nucleic acids play a central role in protein synthesis which is of paramount importance to all tissues of the body, but particularly to those that have a fast turnover like blood. Nucleic acids are also essential in the transmission of hereditary characteristics since they embody the genetic code which itself determines the similarities between offspring and parents. Some of the functions of folic acid are inextricably associated with those of vitamin B_{12} and these will be dealt with under that vitamin.

The causes of folic acid deficiency can vary and some of the more susceptible population groups will now be discussed.

Dietary Considerations

Poor diet combined with destructive cooking methods leads to nutritional folic acid deficiency. Many studies have related deficiency in schoolchildren to dietary intake, for example, it was reported in *Journal of the American Dietetic Association* (1974) that the daily intake of the vitamin was only one-fifth that recommended by the authorities. Elderly people also suffer from folic acid deficiency due mainly to poor eating habits, but their condition is often exacerbated by inefficient absorption of the vitamin from the food. Studies on old people brought into hospital for other reasons showed that 67 per cent of them were folic acid deficient (*British Medical Journal*, 1966); some to such an extent that they were found to have hitherto undetected megaloblastic anaemia.

Pregnancy

The World Health Organization has stated that between one-third and one-half of all pregnant females are deficient in folic acid during the last three months of pregnancy. In many countries regular supplementation with folic acid during pregnancy has eliminated deficiency of the vitamin and the resulting megaloblastic anaemia. It has been estimated in the U.S.A. that needs for the vitamin double during pregnancy.

The foetus is a rapidly growing body and depends on adequate supplies of folic acid which it obtains from the mother's reserves. If these are lacking, the child is as likely to suffer as much as the mother. 'Birth defects are among the grave results of folic acid deficiency in pregnant women' states Dr E. DiCyan, a leading American drug consultant. Deficiency of the vitamin has been associated with some of the complications of pregnancy including toxaemia, premature birth, haemorrhage following birth and the premature separation of the placenta from the uterus (abruptio placentae). The latter condition can lead to a reduction of nutrients to the foetus. Many women with histories of habitual abortion have responded to folic acid supplementation that allows the child to come to full term and normal birth.

Folic Acid and Resistance to Disease
Another effect of receiving decreased amounts of folic acid during foetal development is a lack of resistance to illness in the new-born babe. Although it is only one factor amongst several, folic acid is needed to develop the body's resistance to disease and this functions through the thymus gland which controls the body's immune response. During adulthood, an adequate intake of folic acid is just as important in determining an individual's ability to ward off disease. Conversely, it appears that some patients with bacterial infections are unable to absorb the vitamin from the intestine. This vicious circle can only be broken by injecting the vitamin into the individual.

Folic Acid and the Brain
A study from Massachusetts General Hospital, reported in the *New England Journal of Medicine* (1975), revealed that some mentally disturbed or retarded patients responded favourably to folic acid treatment. Even schizophrenics lost some of their psychotic symptoms. It has been mentioned in Chapter 2 that vitamin B_6 is necessary in the production of certain chemicals that are normally released at nerve endings and folic acid too plays a part in the process. Certainly, in the above-mentioned study, it was found that both vitamin B_6 and folic acid were essential in overcoming the mental symptoms. Neither was effective alone. Yet reports from Northwich Park Hospital, Middlesex have indicated that schizophrenia and other mental conditions have benefited from folic acid alone. What is agreed, however, is that some mental problems will respond to folic acid and at doses of only between 5mg and 20mg per day.

Folic Acid and Medicinal Drugs
Many drugs inhibit the action of folic acid in the body through competitive antagonism. This means that both the

vitamin and the drug compete for the active site on the enzyme responsible for a particular metabolic action. If the vitamin latches onto the enzyme the normal reaction proceeds smoothly. If the drug gets there first, it blocks out the vitamin and the enzyme becomes inactive. Such drugs are similar in chemical structure to folic acid, and so they are readily accepted by the enzyme. Examples are methotrexate used for cancer, immunosuppression (to prevent rejection of transplanted organs) and in psoriasis; pyrimethamine, an antimalarial drug; pentamidine isethionate used to treat parasitic and bacterial infections; trimethoprin which is an antibiotic and the diuretic drug triamterene.

Anti-convulsant drugs are widely used in epilepsy and there are a number of reports that in some individuals they can antagonize the action of folic acid and produce megaloblastic anaemia. Treatment with folic acid is then required to overcome the anaemia, but an excess of the vitamin can neutralize the action of the drug. Such cases are rare, however, and can be controlled by skilled medical treatment.

Other drugs that can cause low folic acid levels in the body are isoniazid – anti-tuberculosis; aspirin in high doses; cholestyramine – anti-cholesterol; and alcohol. Alcohol prevents the absorption of folic acid from the food, inhibits its action in the liver and interferes with its normal action. Oral contraceptives can cause excessive excretion of folic acid sometimes to such an extent that megaloblastic anaemia results.

The Toxicity of Folic Acid

Folic acid is usually well tolerated when taken orally. There have been occasional reports of loss of appetite, nausea, flatulence and abdominal distension when taken at doses of 15mg per day. Sleep disturbances and irritability have been claimed, although some people become overactive. Long-term treatment can precipitate excessive loss of vitamin B_{12} stores. U.K. legislation, however, ensures that high-dose folic acid is not on general sale, so side-effects are not likely to come from self-treatment.

Vitamin B$_{12}$: How it was Isolated

Vitamin B$_{12}$ is the last true vitamin to be discovered despite claims in later years of newer 'vitamins'. Pernicious anaemia (P.A.) first described in 1849, was a killer disease immune to treatment until 1926 when Drs G. R. Minot and W. P. Murphy demonstrated that it could be relieved by whole liver eaten raw. Fortunately for those suffering from the disease, this heroic treatment was eventually replaced by a liver extract that could be injected although, as there was no way of standardizing this extract, results were often variable. The reason that people suffered from this type of anaemia was provided by the classic work of Dr W. B. Castle in 1929, who showed that beef muscle or beef liver when mixed with normal gastric juice and administered to P.A. patients restored normal blood formation. He thus hypothesized the existence of two factors necessary to prevent pernicious anaemia. One was the intrinsic factor present in normal gastric juice; the other was an extrinsic factor present in food. P.A. patients appeared to lack intrinsic factor but the liver extract success suggested that the oral route could be bypassed by injection, so the hunt was on to isolate the extrinsic factor from liver.

Two research groups, one in Britain and one in the U.S.A., succeeded in isolating the new vitamin almost simultaneously in 1948. When it is considered that about 1 tonne of fresh liver yielded only 20mg of the vitamin, the extent of the operation becomes apparent. The vitamin however, is a life-saver for those with pernicious anaemia and an injection of 1mg per month is sufficient to overcome the disease. Although liver is a relatively rich source of the vitamin, it is not a commercial proposition for producing it and fortunately it was soon found that the vitamin was a by-product of bacterial fermentation in the production of antibiotics. Today all vitamin B$_{12}$ is produced from this source, so it can be taken safely by vegetarians and vegans.

The Food Sources of Vitamin B$_{12}$

Vitamin B$_{12}$ is unique amongst the vitamins because it does not occur in plants. It is provided only in foods derived from animals. The bacterial population of the lower intestine can synthesize the vitamin, but it is produced too low down in the gut to be absorbed and used by man. The exception to this is in certain parts of the world where hygiene is not at the same high standard desired elsewhere, with the result that people living there have a bacterial population much higher in the intestine than would be expected. The happy result is that the vitamin produced can be utilized by the body, and the population, despite an almost complete lack of animal products in their diet, do not show any signs of B_{12} deficiency. This ingenious piece of research recently reported from India may go part of the way in explaining why vegans, who partake of no animal foods whatsoever, do not suffer from B_{12} deficiency as often as one would expect from their very limited intake of the vitamin. The levels of vitamin B_{12} in foodstuffs are given in Table 5 (see page 59).

How Vitamin B_{12} Deficiency Develops

In order to absorb vitamin B_{12} it must first be formed into a complex with the intrinsic factor that is produced by the healthy stomach. The complex moves down the gut and is eventually absorbed in the ileum, the lower portion of the small intestine. If the intrinsic factor cannot be produced, vitamin B_{12} cannot be absorbed, so we must regard pernicious anaemia as a disease of malabsorption. Even in a healthy individual, it is unlikely that more than 5 mcg can be absorbed via the intrinsic factor mechanism. This is ample to maintain an adequate supply of vitamin B_{12} in the body. Even when the intrinsic factor is not available, it may take from 6 months to 2 years for the signs of vitamin B_{12} deficiency to show itself. The body does store the vitamin to a certain extent and its requirements are so low that the drain on body reserves is very slow indeed.

If there should be a lack of the intrinsic factor, vitamin B_{12} can only be introduced into the body by intramuscular injection. Claims that sorbitol, for example, can help absorb B_{12} from the food in the absence of this intrinsic factor have never been substantiated. When the intrinsic factor mechanism fails, absorption is by simple diffusion, but never more than 0.9 per cent of an oral dose is assimilated in this way. Even in a healthy individual a 1000mcg oral dose is largely excreted because of the limited absorption powers of the intestine. The only way to introduce large quantities of vitamin B_{12} into the body is by injection into a muscle. Even by this route, different types of vitamin B_{12} vary in their retention by the body. Hydroxocobalamin, for example, is far superior to cyanocobalamin in this respect.

Effects of Vitamin B_{12} Deficiency

Despite the tiny amounts of B_{12} required to maintain health, its deficiency probably affects every cell in the body, but is most severely felt in those tissues where rapid cell division takes place. These are in blood formation and in the lining of the gastro-intestinal tract. The effect on the blood is reflected by the appearance of a megaloblastic anaemia similar to that seen in folic acid deficiency. However, the most insidious and dangerous manifestation of B_{12} deficiency is in the degeneration of the nerve fibres in the spinal cord and elsewhere. In addition to symptoms in the blood and nervous system, deficiency of B_{12} gives rise to smooth sore tongue, menstrual disorders, listlessness, tremors and excessive pigmentation of the hands that, for some unknown reason, only affects coloured people.

How Does Vitamin B_{12} Function?

Vitamin B_{12} is essential to maintain the myelin sheath that surrounds nerves. Myelin is a fatty substance that may be regarded as an insulating cover for nerves in the same way that plastic or rubber is used to insulate electric wires. When the myelin sheath breaks down it is akin to the perishing of electric cable and, in the same way, short circuits may be set up in the nervous system when the inner sensitive parts of the nerve become exposed. Fatty acids are the constituents of myelin and their synthesis is under the direct control of vitamin B_{12}. Lack of the vitamin must, therefore, cause breakdown in the structure of the essential insulator, myelin.

It is impossible to consider the role of vitamin B_{12} in blood formation without reference to the function of folic acid. Both vitamins are required for the synthesis of the constituents of DNA (deoxyribonucleic acid), which is the very basis of body cell production. In the absence of either vitamin, DNA can no longer be synthesized so blood cell production grinds to a halt with the inevitable anaemia as an end-result. Other body processes are also affected, but these relate to one vitamin or the other. It is the blood-forming tissues that reside within the bone marrow that are particularly sensitive to lack of either or both vitamins.

This relationship between folic acid and vitamin B_{12} explains the importance of correct diagnosis and treatment of pernicious anaemia. If a patient has a megaloblastic anaemia that is treated with massive doses of folic acid, the blood picture may revert to normal. However, that anaemia may be due to B_{12} deficiency and it could clear up with these high doses of folic acid, but the nerve degeneration will not be affected. Hence, in the absence of B_{12} treatment, this degeneration will eventually reach the point of no return and the disease will become untreatable.

Vegetarians and particularly vegans are prone to this because in their diet they have high intakes of folic acid and only a marginal intake of vitamin B_{12}. If they are unfortunate enough to suffer from pernicious anaemia, this may be masked by the large intake of folic acid and they are unaware of the disease until nervous symptoms appear.

Therapeutic Uses of Vitamin B_{12}

The knowledge that vitamin B_{12} deficiency produces nerve degeneration has stimulated studies into its use in brain and nerve disturbances. Old people with mild mental problems often respond to the vitamin. Dr O. Abransky of the Hadassah University Medical School of Jerusalem has treated many old people who exhibited mental apathy, moodiness, poor memory, paranoia and confusion with vitamin B_{12} injections, bringing excellent results. A consultant psychiatrist at the University of Aberdeen, Dr J. G. Handerson, has reported similar benefits in old people and believes that 'vitamin B_{12} deficiency may be a possible diagnosis in the majority of psychiatric patients'. Mental disorders due to B_{12} deficiency are not confined to the old, and younger people often benefit from treatment with the vitamin. The fact that mental symptoms often appear before the anaemia associated with B_{12} deficiency would suggest that in these cases the patient's B_{12} status should be first examined. This is particularly so when an adequate intake of the vitamin from the food is in question.

With its discovery, vitamin B_{12} was hailed as the panacea for a wide variety of conditions, but a more sober assessment of its use has rather limited these. There is little doubt, however, that the vitamin can help in the relief of muscle fatigue and in providing extra energy. Simple tiredness was treated with injections of vitamin B_{12} in a study by Drs Ellis and Nasser (*British Journal of Nutrition*, 1973). The criteria assessed were appetite, mood, energy, sleep and an overall feeling of well-being. The vitamin injections were compared with a harmless placebo and neither doctor nor patient knew which was which. In all cases the benefits from the B_{12} were real and unrelated to any psychological effect.

In other respects, vitamin B_{12} appears to potentiate the beneficial effects of folic acid. For example both vitamins are essential in the development of resistance to infection in new-born babes and animals. During pregnancy it is a wise precaution to take both folic acid and B_{12}, according to a report in the *Journal of the American Medical Association* (1972), mainly because of the excessive demands of the foetus. The same group of researchers found that the contraceptive pill can cause over-excretion of both vitamins in those taking it. Supplementation was suggested as the means of overcoming this depletion since the diet is unlikely to provide sufficient vitamins to redress the balance.

How Safe is Vitamin B$_{12}$?

Vitamin B$_{12}$ is probably the safest vitamin known. Very rarely allergic reactions have followed an injection but not from oral administration of the vitamin.

5
OTHER IMPORTANT
B-COMPLEX FACTORS

In this chapter we shall consider four factors that are part of the vitamin B-complex but cannot be regarded as true vitamins for reasons discussed in the Introduction.

Choline: An Anti-fat Agent

Choline is defined as a lipotropic factor which means that it prevents fats from accumulating in the liver by facilitating the transport of those fats to the organs that require them. Liver normally contains only between 5 and 7 per cent of its weight as fat, but in the absence of choline this proportion can increase to as much as 50 per cent. Such fatty deposits, when allowed to build up in the vital organ, adversely affects its normal functioning and the ill-effects are soon felt. There are a number of diseases that can give rise to fatty liver and these include diabetes, alcoholism and protein-deficiency. Lack of choline has been implicated in the development of fatty liver by Dr S. Mookerjea of the University of Toronto, who observed an increase of liver fats during periods of choline deprivation.

When fats are transported from the liver, they do so in the

form of complex substances called phospholipids. These are composed of fats, phosphorus, sugar and choline in combination. According to experimental evidence from animal work published in the *American Journal of Clinical Nutrition* (1965), lack of choline prevented this mechanism from operating with the result that the liver cells soon filled up with unwanted fat. Supplementation with choline not only prevented such changes but actually reversed the process and cleared the liver of accumulated fat. Human studies on infants suffering from fatty liver (*Journal of American Medical Association*, 1951) have confirmed a similar role for choline in human beings.

Why Choline is Essential for Healthy Nerves

Choline is essential to the maintenance of the myelin sheath which, you will recall from Chapter 4, acts as an insulator. In addition to this structural function, however, choline, in the form of a simple derivative called acetylcholine, is essential in transmitting nerve impulses. Although nerves may be thought of as power cables – vehicles for carrying electric impulses – the resemblance ends where the nerve meets another nerve or the muscle it is controlling. Here electrical energy causes acetylcholine, which is stored in the nerve ending, to be released and in so doing it relays the message to the next nerve or to the muscle causing it to react. To prevent the acetylcholine from having a continuous action on the muscle, it is inactivated very quickly allowing the muscle to relax and await the next nerve impulse which starts the whole process over again. Lack of choline means that acetylcholine cannot be produced, so nerve function deteriorates with serious consequences. The therapeutic value of choline in this respect is dealt with later.

Control of Blood Pressure

It is possible that prolonged low levels of choline in the body can give rise to high blood pressure (hypertension). The compound was given to a group of patients suffering from hypertension with beneficial results according to a report in

Journal of Vitaminology (1957). Typical symptoms of palpitations, dizziness and headaches disappeared within two weeks of treatment, together with reduction of the blood pressure to normal. The mechanism of this action is not known, but it could be via the nerves controlling the blood vessels, which in turn determine the blood pressure. Other evidence suggests that low levels of choline throughout life may put some individuals on the road to hypertension in later years.

Choline and Resistance to Disease

We saw in Chapter 4 that folic acid and vitamin B_{12} act together in the development of our resistance to disease. To these vitamins may now be added choline, according to a report from the Massachusetts Institute of Technology in *Science News* (1974). The fourth member of this very important quartet is methionine, an essential amino acid that we obtain from protein in the food.

The link amongst these four is that they are all concerned with the transfer of methyl groups – simple entities that are the basis of many of life's processes. Introduction of a methyl group into various compounds enables them to participate in the many body functions required for health e.g. RNA and DNA transformations. Lack of any one of these components in a pregnant animal deprives the offspring of the ability to ward off infection after birth. An ample supply of methyl groups is essential for growth of the foetus and particularly the thymus gland which is at the centre of the body's immune response. Deficiency of choline in the mother leads to smaller and less well-developed thymus glands in the offspring, with consequent lower resistance to disease. It may be significant in this respect that human breast milk is far richer in choline than cow's milk, which may explain in part the current belief that breast-fed babies have apparently a better developed immunity system.

Where Do We Obtain Choline?

Choline is widely distributed in plants and animals and the richest sources include brewer's yeast, fish, soybeans, nuts, liver, eggs, and wheatgerm. Choline usually occurs as a component of phospholipids, that are complexes of fatty acids, phosphorus, sugar and choline. The most abundant phospholipid is lecithin and this represents one of the richest sources of choline. There have been some measurements of choline in foods and these include: egg yolk, 1700mg per 100g (there is none in egg-white); meat, 600mg per 100g; cereals, 100mg per 100g; desiccated liver, 2000mg per 100g; brewer's yeast, 300mg per 100g; and pure lecithin, which contains an average of 3430mg per 100g. Daily intake from an average diet has been calculated as between 500mg and 1000mg. The significance of the daily requirements is obscure since the body is probably capable of synthesizing its needs from other food materials. However, there are examples of complaints that have responded to extra choline in the diet which suggests that body synthesis may not always be sufficient.

Diseases of Fat Metabolism

The role of choline in ensuring mobility of fat and maintaining it in solution has lead to its use in diseases where fat metabolism has gone wrong. In the *Proceedings of the Society of Biology and Medicine* (1950), Drs L. M. Morrison and W. F. Gonzalez reported beneficial effects of choline treatment in patients suffering from atherosclerosis – a condition where the blood vessels become thickened by the deposition of fat. In the form of lecithin, choline has also been used successfully in those suffering from angina, thrombosis and stroke. Any condition that may be related to a high blood cholesterol and fat content is often helped by choline supplementation. It must be stressed, however, that choline is usually given in the form of lecithin in these cases. This is because lecithin also contains unsaturated fatty acids which contribute to the beneficial action of choline in any upset of fat metabolism.

Senile Dementia

A very recent development in the treatment of senile dementia is the use of choline as a simple dietary supplement in the form of lecithin. Experimental studies by Drs M. J. Hirsch and R. J. Wurtman from the Massachusetts Institute of Technology showed that consumption of a single meal containing lecithin increased the levels of choline and its product acetylcholine in the brain of rats. Since acetylcholine is essential as a chemical transmitter in brain functioning, it seemed logical to try choline as a supplement in those conditions in man where acetylcholine may be deficient.

In a number of pilot studies this has been carried out on patients suffering from mental deterioration, with promising results. A typical trial was reported from Canada (*The Lancet*, 1978) when a dose of 25g of lecithin per day (i.e. 900mg choline) produced dramatic improvement in these patients. The treatment is a simple dietary one and is without side-effects at the dose of 25g lecithin per day. What did emerge was that lecithin is preferable to choline as a food supplement. Choline is better absorbed as lecithin and there are more chances of side-effects when choline itself is taken in high doses.

Inositol: A Fat-Fighter

We have seen above how important choline is as a lipotropic agent in ensuring that fat is kept in solution and is not deposited in the wrong places in the body. The second factor that also has this property is inositol, but it is structurally very different from choline and hence exerts its lipotropic action in a different way. The fat-fighting properties of inositol appear to act in addition to those associated with choline, so it is not surprising that both are essential in controlling fat metabolism. There are reports from the *American Heart Journal*, 1949, by Drs I. Leinwand and D. H. Moore that giving 3g of inositol daily to atherosclerotic patients resulted in a reduction of blood fats and cholesterol. Similar treatment reduced the excessive deposition of fat in those suffering from fatty liver. Despite these early reports, however, it is now accepted that the best way to restore fat metabolism to normal is by treating with both choline and inositol. Drs D. A. Sherber and M. M. Levites reported in the *Journal of the American Medical Association* in 1953 that this approach was successful in reducing cholesterol levels in all their patients subjected to the treatment.

Effects of Inositol on the Nervous System

The brain and spinal cord nerves contain very high concentrations of inositol. Part of this is found in the myelin sheath, as with choline, but inositol appears to have some function not associated with its structural property. Thus Dr C. C. Pfeiffer at the Brain Bio Centre, Princeton, New Jersey, has studied the effect of inositol on brain wave patterns in schizophrenics and normal people. He claims that inositol has a similar anti-anxiety effect to that of librium or meprobamate (e.g. Equagesic, Miltown). The calming effect of inositol can thus make it a possible alternative to the widely-prescribed librium and meprobamate. In this respect it is attractive to speculate that perhaps anxiety, irritability and hyperactivity may be related to a lack of inositol in the brain or some simple block in its metabolism.

All cells in the body appear to need inositol to stay healthy, but it is especially necessary for the bone marrow, eye membranes and the cells lining the gastro-intestinal tract. Unsubstantiated reports claim that it is food for stimulating good hair growth and overcoming baldness. These properties may be related to the role of inositol in maintaining cell structure in a healthy state.

Sources of Inositol

The compound is widely distributed in plants and animals with the richest sources recognized as beef brain, beef heart, wheatgerm, wholegrains, brown rice, nuts, brewer's yeast and citrus fruits. Some measurements are given in Table 6. Cereals and vegetables do not contain inositol as such, but as a derivative known as phytic acid. This is simply inositol

Table 6. Choline and Inositol Contents of Raw Foods

Food Item	Choline (mg per 100g)	Inositol (mg per 100g)
Liver	650	340
Desiccated liver	2170	1100
Beef steak	600	260
Beef heart	1720	1600
Veal	40	30
Chicken	60	50
Fish (white)	20	20
Fish (fatty)	40	20
Shellfish	50	40
Eggs (yolk)	1700	20
Milk (cows)	11	20
Cheese (hard)	12	20
Yogurt	10	15
Wholemeal bread	80	100
White bread	54	75
Wheatgerm	505	690
Wheat grains	155	190
Oatflakes	240	320
Maize (corn)	100	50
Soya flour (full fat)	70	70
Citrus fruits (peeled)	85	210
Bananas	44	120
Nuts (fresh)	220	180
Nuts (roasted)	220	180
Potatoes	20	30
Root vegetables (carrots etc.)	40	50
Greenleaf vegetables	80	100
Pulses (beans, peas etc.)	120	160
Yeast (brewer's, dried)	300	50
Lecithin granules	3430	2857
Lecithin oil	800	360

complexed with phosphate, but phytic acid has properties far removed from those of inositol. For example, it complexes some minerals such as zinc, iron and calcium making them unavailable for absorption. Free inositol on the other hand can actually increase absorption of some minerals. Some phytic acid is eventually degraded to give inositol, but the extent of this is not known. Suffice to say, however, that there is ample free inositol in a good diet to ensure there is no deficiency. Added to this is the fact that both body cells and intestinal bacteria are able to convert glucose to inositol so a deficiency of the compound appears highly unlikely in a healthy individual.

The Best Inositol Supplement
Lecithin supplies inositol as well as choline, and in a similar amount. In fact, it is highly likely that the anti-fat actions of choline and inositol reside in their presence in the lecithin molecule. With ample supplies of choline and inositol in the food, the body is capable of incorporating both of them into lecithin. Similarly, it can utilize both compounds when they are fed as lecithin. It is likely that, to obtain the maximum benefit, at least as far as their fat-fighting qualities are concerned, the lecithin should be from plant sources e.g. soya.

Daily intakes of inositol are probably similar to those of choline within the range 500 to 1000mg. Therapeutic doses can go higher than this with no fear of side-effects. It is preferable to take inositol as plant lecithin because of the beneficial effects of the accompanying choline and unsaturated fatty acids.

Para-aminobenzoic Acid (PABA): The Cosmetic Factor
The compound para-aminobenzoic acid had been known to chemists for many years before its importance in nutrition was discovered. As with other members of the B-complex, its relationship to bacterial function was investigated long before there was any clue to its possible use in animals. Professor D. D. Woods, working at Oxford University, had

observed that PABA was essential to the growth of bacteria. Any agent that denied the micro-organisms this essential nutrient prevented their growth and hence helped to overcome the infection that they caused. Such agents were found to be the sulphonamide drugs which are so similar in structure to PABA that they were able to block the action of the vitamin by competitive antagonism (compare folic acid in Chapter 4). This early use of growth-factor antagonists to destroy bacteria paved the way for the development of many of the antibiotics in use today.

Although PABA is undoubtedly a growth factor or vitamin for micro-organisms, there is no hard evidence that it is one for man. If it was, sulphonamides could not be used safely, as they would also deprive the treated person of PABA. What is established is that PABA is present as part of the chemical structure of folic acid, one of the B vitamins. It must be stressed that this does not mean that by taking PABA the body itself is able to convert it to folic acid. What may happen is that the bacteria that inhabit the lower part of the gut are able to utilize the compound in production of the vitamin. Whether this source of folic acid can be absorbed and used by the body is, however, highly debatable.

PABA in Animals

In animal experiments there is evidence that PABA is essential in the production of body protein. In addition, it appears to be a necessary factor for normal synthesis of red blood cells. It is highly likely that PABA helps in these functions through its conversion first to folic acid which performs similar actions in man. Whether PABA is a vitamin in its own right is, therefore, controversial. There is no doubt, however, that a sign of PABA deficiency in animals is premature greying of hair. Supplementing the diet with the factor restores the hair colour to normal. Despite many attempts to utilize PABA in restoring the natural colour to grey-haired persons, however, there is no evidence that it can do so in man.

PABA in Man

The only beneficial effects of PABA in man relate to its action on the skin. One particular complaint is vitiligo which has defied medical treatment for many years. Vitiligo affects mainly young people and it is characterized by the sudden appearance of light areas on the skin, particularly in places exposed to sunlight. These areas appear to be incapable of producing the normal skin pigment known as melanin. The condition does not cause any physical ill-effects, but it can be mentally disturbing because of its appearance. The usual treatment is to hide the blemishes with cosmetics, although occasionally corticosteroid creams have been used with limited success.

A clinical trial carried out in 1943 and reported in *Archives of Dermatology* by Dr M. J. Costello produced promising results on the treatment of vitiligo with PABA. These led in turn to more comprehensive trials by Dr B. Sieve at Tufts Medical School, U.S.A. The subjects, both male and female, of ages from 10 to 70 years, were injected with a long-acting preparation of PABA in a potency of 50mg twice per day. In addition, a 100mg tablet of the compound was taken orally twice per day in between the injections. After two weeks new, light-coloured pigmentation appeared in the affected areas. Steady improvement continued over the next 14 weeks with the slow appearance of darker pigments resulting in normal colouring after six to eight months. It is not likely that vitiligo is due simply to deficiency of PABA and more recent studies of Dr C. C. Pfeiffer at the Brain Bio Centre, Princeton suggests that in addition to this factor, pantothenic acid, vitamin B_6, zinc and manganese should also be taken in good amounts.

PABA as a Sunscreen Agent

Sunburn and suntan are caused by the ultraviolet light (UV) in the sun's rays, and because UV light is not visible, its burning and tanning effects are not necessarily related to brightness. Light is defined by its wavelength and it has been established that UV light, with a wavelength below

320nm (nanometres) causes burning but not tanning. UV light of greater wavelength gives rise to tanning without burning. An effective sunscreen agent must therefore screen out and absorb light of wavelength less than 320nm. PABA is such an agent when applied to the skin.

An evaluation of 24 sunscreen agents in desert, temperate and alpine conditions indicated that 5 per cent PABA in aqueous alcohol is the best protectant for the skin. According to this report from Harvard University in the *New England Journal of Medicine* (1969), PABA actually enters the skin layers and reacts with them producing a long-term protective effect unlike the commercial synthetic products that are removed by bathing. There have been no cases of sensitivity of the skin caused by PABA.

Recent studies on mice, reported from the University of Miami, have looked at the protective action of PABA against cancer of the skin. These mice are bred hairless and are thus prone to skin cancer induced by UV light. Pre-treating their skin with PABA prevented the development of tumours, even in the presence of chemicals that are known to give rise to cancer under the influence of UV light. With our present knowledge that over-exposure to UV light can cause skin cancer in fair-skinned populations of the world, it would appear to be a sensible precaution for these people to protect themselves with properly applied solutions of PABA when they expose themselves to the sun.

Food Sources of PABA

PABA occurs in food as a member of the B-complex and so it is present wherever this is to be found. Thus the richest sources are liver, eggs, molasses, brewer's yeast and wheat-germ. Few quantitative measurements have been made, but it is known that baker's yeast may contain from 5 to 6mg per kilogram and brewer's yeast from 10 to 100mg per kilogram of yeast.

How Safe is PABA?

PABA is usually well tolerated in low doses, but high intakes can give rise to nausea, vomiting, itch, skin rash and liver damage. Obviously, because of the antagonism mentioned previously, it should not be taken by those on sulphonamides treatment. It is for these reasons that a limit of 30mg per tablet has been imposed by the health authorities in the U.K.

Orotic Acid: The Milk Factor

During the early 1950s there was renewed interest in the basic body constituents, RNA (ribonucleic acids) and DNA (deoxyribonucleic acids). It was realized that the processes of cell regeneration, repair and growth were dependent upon and controlled by these compounds and in them also lay the secret of heredity. As with much of the previous research on other members of the B-complex, it was found that in micro-organisms one particular compound held a central role in the synthesis of the constituents that made up the RNA and DNA. This was designated vitamin B_{13} known also by the trivial name of orotic acid. Its importance was reflected in the finding that it lay as an intermediate on the pathway of synthesis of RNA and DNA. Hence, micro-organisms deprived of it failed to multiply and eventually died. Orotic acid is therefore a growth factor for certain bacteria. The richest source is liquid whey and it was from this that the factor was eventually isolated. Hopes that orotic acid would prove to be a new vitamin for animals and man were also dashed when it was found that the body was perfectly capable of making all its needs from precursors readily available from the diet, either directly or indirectly. This in no way diminishes the importance of orotic acid in animals as it still occupies a central role in the production of animal RNA and DNA. However, it satisfied none of the criteria to justify calling it a vitamin, even though it has been claimed to have beneficial effects in certain diseases. The only rich source of orotic acid other than liquid whey is root vegetables, although as a member of the B-complex it appears in tiny amounts wherever the complex is found.

Remedial Properties of Orotic Acid

Conditions claimed to have been helped by orotic acid include multiple sclerosis. Dr J. Evers, from West Germany, reported in *Cancer Control Journal* (1971) that injections of orotic acid had been successful in treating multiple sclerosis in some patients. The relationship between nutrition and multiple sclerosis is highly complex and many regimes of supplementation with vitamins and minerals along with diets with certain ingredients removed have been tried with varying success. Perhaps orotic acid may help in some cases, but it may be of significance that other reports have not followed those of Dr Evers in later years.

When we consider the central role of orotic acid in body cell regeneration perhaps it is not surprising that it may help in inflammatory conditions. Dr H. A. Nieper, who has pioneered much of the clinical studies on orotic acid, claims that cases of chronic hepatitis (some including cirrhosis of the liver) responded to orotic acid in the form of calcium orotate. Treatment ranged over 6 to 18 months during which time the hepatitis was cured and the cirrhosis condition was prevented from developing further. The successful treatment of gout with orotic acid has been reported in the *Journal of Annals of Rheumatic Diseases* (1966). Gout is caused by an upset in the metabolism of RNA and DNA that leads to overproduction of a compound called uric acid in the blood. Uric acid is not very soluble and when present in excess it tends to be deposited in the joints as crystals leading to the intense pain associated with the condition. In the report four patients were given 4g of orotic acid for six days with great improvement. The compound in some way stimulated the dissolution and excretion of uric acid, so removing the cause of the complaint.

Mineral Salts of Orotic Acid

There have been many reports of clinical success using specific mineral salts of orotic acid in such diverse conditions as decalcification of bones, muscle cramps, nervous disorders, arteriosclerosis, overweight, angina, arthritis and

cancer. Careful consideration of the evidence strongly
suggests that the benefits in these complaints are related
more to the mineral component than to the orotic acid.
There is no convincing evidence that orotic acid is acting
other than as a simple carrier of minerals akin to the citrates,
fumarates, aspartates, gluconates and sulphates already in
common use in medicine.

It is impossible to suggest a daily requirement of orotic
acid as the body is apparently able to synthesize all that it
needs. It is generally considered harmless when given as the
free compound orotic acid. For example, up to 4g per day
by mouth caused no harm over many days of treatment. On
the other hand, the mineral complexes calcium orotate and
magnesium orotate may cause an unpleasant sensation in
the mouth often coupled with a heat reaction in the limbs
and head.

6

THE THERAPEUTIC FACTORS: PANGAMIC ACID AND LAETRILE

Pangamic acid was discovered by the father and son team Drs E. T. Krebs and E. T. Krebs Jr in 1951 when they isolated a new crystalline water-soluble factor from apricot kernels. Further studies indicated that the new factor was widely distributed in plants and particularly seeds, so it was named pangamic acid from the Greek words 'pan', meaning 'everywhere' and 'gami', meaning 'family'. Its association with the B-complex led to the designation vitamin B_{15}, but it has never been proved to satisfy the criteria for vitamin status so it is more correctly termed the B_{15} factor or, preferably, pangamic acid.

Since its discovery in the U.S.A., pangamic acid has had a chequered career. Although there was almost total disinterest in the country in which it was first discovered, it was eagerly investigated by the Russians who undertook a vast amount of research into its properties and medical application. Now researchers in Western Europe and the U.S.A. are looking anew at B_{15} some thirty years after its discovery. Pangamic acid occurs in rice bran, rice polishings, brewer's yeast, cow's blood and horse liver, as well as in seeds. The quantities present in foodstuffs are given in Table 7. These are the amounts in unprocessed foods. Like other members of the B-complex, B_{15} is lost during food processing and refining and, unlike some vitamins, it is not replaced. In supplement form it is offered as sodium or calcium pangamate as these are the stable forms of the factor.

Table 7. Pangamic Acid Content of Raw Foods

Food Item	B_{15} – Pangamic Acid (mg per 100g)
Liver (pig)	22
Wholemeal flour	8
Wheat bran	31
Wheatgerm	70
Oatflakes	106
Maize (corn)	150
Rice bran	200
Barley	12
Yeast (brewer's, dried)	128

The Function of Pangamic Acid
Most of the power of B_{15} lies in its function as an agent which stimulates the carriage of oxygen to the blood from the lungs and from the blood to the muscles and vital organs. It is for these reasons that B_{15} is popular amongst athletes, but the same properties make the factor a valuable adjunct in the treatment of various complaints. Diseases once associated with ageing, such as angina (insufficient oxygen to the heart), stroke (insufficient oxygen to the brain) and senility, are relieved by B_{15} because of its ability to increase the blood supply to the appropriate organ.

Tiredness and exhaustion can be a direct result of

inefficient transfer of oxygen from blood to muscles and it is here that pangamic acid is able to increase the supply of this essential energizer. In fact, the Russians established in *Reports of the Academy of Sciences* (1962) that hypoxia – insufficient oxygen supply – is treated most efficiently with B_{15}, and they use the factor in the form of calcium pangamate routinely in any surgery involving the heart or blood system.

The second property possessed by pangamic acid is that of a lipotropic agent. We saw in Chapter 5 that choline, another member of the B-complex, and methionine, an amino acid, share this facility. Like these, pangamic acid is a methyl donor, which simply means that by passing a methyl group to certain substances in the liver and other organs it is able to ensure normal fat metabolism and prevent fat being deposited in the wrong places. The ability to donate methyl groups confers on pangamic acid an important protective role. Poisonous substances that enter the body are rendered harmless by the transfer to them of methyl groups from pangamic acid. Free radicals, which are toxic substances produced by the body's own processes, are usually disposed of by conversion to harmless compounds by reaction with methyl groups. In a healthy individual this represents no problem, but if the supply of the detoxifying methyl groups dries up, poisons can build up within the body. This is probably one of the contributory facts in the process of ageing, hence the claims that pangamic acid can help repair the ravages of time.

The third function attributed to pangamic acid is its stimulant effect on the glands of the body that produce anti-stress hormones. You will recall in Chapter 3 that the B-complex vitamins pantothenic acid and biotin exert a similar influence because they are necessary cofactors in making these hormones. It is not known by which mechanism pangamic acid helps, but measurements of blood hormone levels after B_{15} treatment have indicated an increase in concentration. This property also makes a useful contribution to the beneficial effects of the factor in athletes.

These people are under both physical and mental stress thanks to their muscular exertion and the strain of competition, so pangamic acid can help on both counts.

Some examples of the therapeutic value of pangamic acid will now be discussed.

Pangamic Acid in Heart Disease

Professor Y. Y. Shpirt and his colleagues at various Moscow clinics have tested pangamic acid in patients recovering from coronary thrombosis and in others with high blood pressure. The regime used was to give calcium pangamate orally in doses of 20mg or 40mg three times per day. All patients were closely monitored and assessed in terms of disappearance of heart pain and improvement in breathing. Out of 118 cases there were good results observed in 49 patients with a satisfactory response in 55. Eleven of them showed no improvement with only 3 indicating slight deterioration. Although less than 50 per cent (i.e. 49) of the patients were actually relieved of the symptoms mentioned, the results are promising as the age groups were from 68 to 82 years and the trial was continued for only 30 days maximum.

Use in Atherosclerosis of the Heart

Atherosclerosis is a thickening of the inside wall of blood vessels due to laying down of fatty deposits. It is due to an upset in fat and cholesterol metabolism and the resulting narrowed blood vessels decrease the oxygen supply to the heart. When 57 patients suffering from the disease were treated with pangamic acid at the same Moscow clinics as in the first trial and at the same dosage, results were rather more promising. The number of cases responding well was 26, whilst 22 were satisfactory and there was either no effect at all or deterioration in the remaining 9. Those who responded reported an improvement in general well-being, cheerfulness, disappearance of headaches, improvement of sleep and alleviation of pain around the heart and decreased breathlessness. These promising results were considered to

a direct beneficial action of pangamic acid on
al fat metabolism and increased blood supply
oxygen) to the heart muscle.

Bronchial Asthma

In a trial organized by Drs N. I. Pressman and D. G.
Opalinskaya in Moscow hospitals, pangamic acid was given
to asthmatic patients in two ways. For up to 30 days they
were given oral doses of between 120 and 160mg per day
plus 80mg per day given by aerosol directly into the
bronchii and lungs. This is now a standard mode of
applying many drugs to asthmatics. A high positive response
was obtained with 14 out of 17 patients relieved of the
breathlessness and outright attacks associated with the
complaint. What was particularly gratifying was that these
people had not responded to conventional anti-asthmatic
drugs previously given. The authors admit however that
response is better in those suffering from the milder forms
of asthma.

Atherosclerosis of the Lower Limbs

Narrowing of the arteries supplying blood to the legs and
feet results in the inability of the individual to walk very far
without intense pain developing in the lower limbs, due
mainly to deprivation of oxygen to the muscles. The effect of
calcium pangamate in daily doses of 120 to 150mg for up to
30 days was studied in patients suffering from the condition.
In addition, vitamins A (7500 i.u.) and E (100 i.u.) were
given as a supplement. A total of 15 out of 27 patients
undergoing this treatment demonstrated a good response –
they found that their pain disappeared and that they were
able to walk much further distances. This report from the
U.S.S.R. Public Health Ministry was mainly on people
suffering from the early stages of the disease, but it was
followed up by later studies showing that, even in the more
advanced cases, benefit can be expected from the calcium
pangamate plus vitamin treatment. In these patients, however, intramuscular injection of pangamic acid and the
vitamins produced better results.

Diabetes

Clinical experiments carried out on calcium pangamate had indicated a clear role for the factor in controlling sugar metabolism in diabetic rats. At the same time it is now well established that complications induced by long-term diabetes include atherosclerosis, coronary arteriosclerosis and eventually gangrene of the lower limbs. There was thus the possibility that pangamic acid could help the diabetic on two counts; first, by reducing the blood sugar and second, by improving the blood supply to all parts of the body.

Studies were therefore instituted by Dr O. L. Bobrava at the Polyclinic of the U.S.S.R. Public Health Ministry on how calcium pangamate might benefit diabetes. The results were very promising but, at present, are still very much in the preliminary stage. Calcium pangamate was given orally in a dose of 50mg three times per day to those suffering from diabetes with and without gangrene. A constant feature was a steady reduction in blood sugar to normal levels when the disease had been previously treated by diet only. For those on insulin injections or an oral drug treatment, it was possible to reduce the quantity of either drug when on calcium pangamate treatment and still keep the blood sugar down to normal levels. It must be stressed though that calcium pangamate cannot replace insulin and oral hypoglycaemic drugs, but simply complements their action. Whenever gangrenous symptoms associated with the diabetes were present, the Russians found that these too were reduced on calcium pangamate therapy. It is too early to suggest that calcium pangamate can help in all cases of diabetes and such treatment should be under medical supervision anyway. However, there is no doubt that this B-complex factor shows promising potential and it is to be hoped that larger scale clinical trials in diabetes should settle the role of pangamic acid in the treatment of this condition once and for all.

Doses of pangamic acid up to 300mg per day appear to be safe in human beings. Occasionally a transient flushing of the skin occurs, probably associated with a mild dilatory action on the capillaries. Calcium pangamate appears to be tolerated more than sodium pangamate.

Laetrile – B$_{17}$

No other member of the B-complex is calculated to cause more controversy in medical and lay circles as B$_{17}$, known also as laetrile, a contracted name for the tongue twisting compound *lae*vo-mandeloni*trile*-beta glucuronoside. This member of the B-complex, like B$_{15}$, was revealed by the research of the Drs E. T. Krebs in the early 1950s, although laetrile strictly speaking is derived from the naturally occurring substance called amygdalin. The reasons for the controversy lies in the claim that here is a cure for cancer.

Laetrile from Amygdalin

Amygdalin has been known as a constituent of seeds and kernels for over a century and it has been used in cancer therapy since 1845. No concrete evidence of its effectiveness resulted from this use, mainly because controlled clinical trials as we know them today were unheard of then. Nevertheless, before the advent of chemotherapy for cancer, amygdalin was in wide use and there is little doubt that, in some cases, it must have helped in controlling the condition and, perhaps, sometimes even curing it. The richest sources of amygdalin are bitter almonds, and the kernels of apricot and peach seeds. Laetrile, which is related to and can also be derived from amygdalin, is its synthetic counterpart and is the actual material used to treat cancer. For the purposes of this book, however, both compounds should be regarded as synonymous.

The naturally occurring amygdalin, which is present in apricot kernels, and the synthetic laetrile, which is not generally available, are defined as nitrilosides. Nitriloside means cyanide-containing and it is the presence of this poison that is alleged to confer on laetrile its anti-cancer properties. Cyanide in various forms is present in many of our foodstuffs, among which are cassava, sweet potato, yam, maize, millet, sugar cane, peas and beans (particularly lima and butter). The kernels of almond, lemon, lime, apple, pear, cherry, apricot, prune and plum, perhaps not regarded as usual food items today, are all rich sources of cyanide.

A good diet will naturally provide a few milligrams of cyanide per day, but only in an organically-bound form that is harmless until the cyanide is liberated as hydrogen cyanide. This potential poison is liberated by an enzyme called beta-glucosidase which is widely distributed in low concentrations throughout the body tissues. There is no cause for alarm in this fact because the body has a very efficient mechanism for disposing of hydrogen cyanide in these small amounts: an enzyme called rhodanese, that is widely distributed throughout the body, neatly converts hydrogen cyanide into harmless substances that the body can make use of. Hence, in a normal individual, a balance exists between the two enzymes, one of which is producing hydrogen cyanide in small amounts and the other is destroying it.

How these Mechanisms Relate to Cancer

The whole concept of cancer therapy with laetrile depends upon two facts. First, cancer cells are rich in the cyanide-producing enzyme beta-glucosidase and second, cancer cells are devoid of the cyanide-destroying enzyme rhodanese. Hence, the argument goes, cancer cells are unique because they stimulate the conversion of nitrilosides to hydrogen cyanide, but are incapable of defending themselves against the poison. So, in the presence of nitrilosides the cells would regress and die. Hydrogen cyanide is not the only poison produced by the enzymatic breakdown of laetrile. Benzaldehyde, the material that gives bitter almonds their characteristic smell, is also formed. Dr E. T. Krebs, working with mice who had developed cancers, discovered that although either hydrogen cyanide or benzaldehyde was capable of destroying cancer cells, the combination was far more lethal than the expected additive effect. In fact, both compounds are synergistic and this gives added impetus to the anti-cancer role of laetrile.

Dietary Evidence for the Benefits of Laetrile

A study of the dietary habits of an isolated community can be indicative of the role of foods in maintaining health, but it does not represent absolute proof. However, there are a number of various groups of people throughout the world who are virtually cancer-free and one of the most studied of these is the Hunzakuts in the Kingdom of Hunza. The area lies in the Himalayan Mountains and its inhabitants are renowned for their longevity. They are also noted for their natural way of life which includes a diet that must be regarded as well-nigh perfect. One of the prime features of this diet is a high intake of foods containing nitrilosides, among which the most highly prized are apricots. Unlike those in the West, however, the Hunzakuts eat the flesh of the fruit plus the kernel of the stone. It has been calculated that their daily intake of these nitrilosides is some 200 times that of an average Western diet. Apricots grow abundantly in the area and are a staple feature of their diet throughout the year. Cancer is unknown in Hunza, despite an average lifespan of over 80 years.

Dr R. McCarrison, Director of Nutrition Research in India, was so impressed with these observations that he compared the cancer-inducing properties of various national diets with that of the Hunzakuts in experimental animals. Indian, Pakistani, British and American diets caused many diseases amongst the animals associated with the heart, the liver, the kidneys and the gastro-intestinal system and, of course, these included various types of cancers. Those on the Hunza diet remained free of all complaints.

Two other groups of people untouched by 'civilization' were the Eskimos and the North American Indians who have been studied before and after being introduced to Western-type diets. In their traditional way of life Eskimos subsisted on food that is a good source of nitrilosides. They eat salads composed of amygdalin-rich grasses and berries. Even the meat from caribou and other grazing animals is rich in these compounds because these beasts live on foliage abundant with nitrilosides. Fortunately, these cyanide-

containing compounds which act like laetrile are stable and
survive the drying processes used to preserve the foods. This
ensured a high intake of these useful substances throughout
the year in the Eskimo's diet. Perhaps this is why these
people were virtually cancer-free.

Studies on the American Indians reported in the *Journal of
the American Medical Association* (1949) concluded that these
people too were almost cancer-free while they lived on their
traditional diets. The incidence of malignant cancer was
only 36 cases out of 30,000 admissions to the Granada
Arizona Mission Hospital. In a comparable white American
population there would have been 1800 patients with
malignant growths. Analysis of the diet of these Indians
revealed a high intake of nitrilosides per day, including in
some cases as much as 8000 mg.

What is revealing, although particularly tragic, is that
whenever these groups of people take up the Western way of
life and its dietary habits, within two generations they suffer
from the same diseases at the same incidence as the
indigenous population. Although a change in eating habits
is only one factor involved in their new mode of living, it
must make a major contribution to the increased risks of
developing certain diseases, among which is cancer.

Laetrile and Cancer Treatment

Cancer is an emotive subject and its treatment with laetrile
has provoked many bitter arguments. Numerous books
have been written on the subject, most of them presenting
case histories of those who responded to laetrile treatment.
These mainly originated in the U.S.A. where, despite
legislation to prevent its use, laetrile is widely prescribed by
some doctors with a certain amount of success. Most of the
evidence therefore comes from clandestine treatments, but
the very nature of these makes doctors unwilling to reveal
their results and it becomes impossible to assess the therapy
on a firm basis.

In an attempt to find out just how successful laetrile
treatment is, a survey was carried out in the U.S.A. recently

when those treated with the factor were asked to supply details of their response. A group of 60,000 people were solicited and only 93 replies were received. Of these merely 22 cases could be evaluated of which six validated the claim that the patient improved while taking laetrile. This is typical of the clumsy approach that the authorities have made in trying to assess laetrile in retrospect, but at least it had one successful outcome. The fact that six people had improved was sufficient to warrant a properly-conducted clinical trial on laetrile and this was something that had been previously denied. The clinical trial is now in progress, but as yet no preliminary results are available.

One of the problems associated with laetrile treatment is that of dosage. The isolated compound can be measured and given to the patient like any other drug. When using powdered seeds or kernels, however, it is not so easy to determine how much amygdalin is present. Apricot kernels for example contain about 5mg of B_{17} per kernel, but this is simply an average and can sometimes be six times that figure. Dr E. T. Krebs has suggested a minimum daily intake to maintain health of 50mg B_{17} which would be supplied by 10 to 12 apricot kernels per day, assuming an average content of 4-5mg per kernel. However, treatment of cancer with laetrile requires much more. Moreover, the material is better injected, particularly during the early part of the treatment. The only way, therefore, to assess a meaningful dose of B_{17} is to use standardized laetrile. For these reasons self-medication with the material cannot be recommended. Ground-up apricot seeds should be regarded as a dietary supplement that supplies dietary needs rather than as a therapeutic treatment.

An American physician, Dr John Richardson has claimed success with laetrile treatment of cancer in his book *Laetrile Case Histories* (1977) published by American Media, P.O. Box 4646, Westlake Village, California, 91359*. Treatment is not confined to laetrile but includes a sensible diet, pancreatic enzyme tablets, pangamic acid (B_{15}), vitamin C in high dose, amino acid tablets, chelated minerals, vitamins with a high intake of vitamin E plus extra protein. Laetrile is given in doses of between 3g and 9g intravenously or intramuscularly along with 1g taken in tablet form. Treatment has continued for 18 months or longer. Dr Richardson emphasizes that laetrile therapy is not given alone but is an adjunct to a whole new dietary regime. For these reasons and by virtue of the necessity for injection of laetrile, such treatments are in the province of the practitioner and are not suitable for self-medication.

How safe is Laetrile?

The fact that laetrile contains cyanide makes it extremely important that anyone who is on the treatment is regularly monitored for symptoms of cyanide poisoning. A typical case was described in the *New England Journal of Medicine* (1979). A female of 48 suffering from lung cancer was being treated with laetrile orally and by injection. After a 9-day course she complained of cold sweats, headaches, nausea, lethargy and breathlessness. Her blood pressure was very low. The level of cyanide in her blood was near lethal limits. Treatment with anti-cyanide substances restored her to her pre-laetrile condition. This case is quoted because it is important to realize that laetrile in therapeutic doses is not as safe as its protagonists would like to believe. There are claims in the medical literature that 17 patients have died from cyanide poisoning brought on by excessive laetrile intake. These facts illustrate the importance of ensuring that treatment with B_{17} is carried out under medical supervision and monitoring.

*For further reading see also *About Laetrile* and *An End to Cancer?*, both by Leon Chaitow and published by Thorsons Publishers Limited, Denington Estate, Wellingborough, Northants.

INDEX